NEPHROLOGY RESEARCH AND CLINICAL DEVELOPMENTS

URIC ACID

DETECTION, APPLICATIONS AND ROLE IN HEALTH AND DISEASE

Nephrology Research and Clinical Developments

Additional books in this series can be found on Nova's website under the Series tab.

Additional e-books in this series can be found on Nova's website under the eBook tab.

NEPHROLOGY RESEARCH AND CLINICAL DEVELOPMENTS

URIC ACID

DETECTION, APPLICATIONS AND ROLE IN HEALTH AND DISEASE

MARY NEWMAN
EDITOR

NOVA BIOMEDICAL
New York

Library of Congress Cataloging-in-Publication Data

Library of Congress Control Number: 2016954744
ISBN: 978-1-53610-287-1

Published by Nova Science Publishers, Inc. † New York

CONTENTS

PREFACE

Uric acid (UA) is an end-product of purine derivatives in human metabolism. Without further metabolism, it is excreted by kidneys and intestinal tract. Its serum concentration is controlled by the balance between production and excretion. High concentration of UA in human body has been discovered to be associated with various diseases, such as gout, hyperuricaemia, Lesch-Nyan disease, obesity, diabetes, high cholesterol, hypertension, kidney disease and heart disease. This book discusses the detection, applications and role in health and disease of uric acid.

Chapter 1 - Uric acid (2,4,6-trihydroxypurine) (UA) is an end-product of purine derivatives in human metabolism. Excessive amount of it in serum is known as hyperuricemia and has been found to be related to hypertension, metabolic syndrome and cardiovascular disease. Therefore, fast and reliable detection of UA content in biological fluids is conventionally demanded for disease diagnosis and treatment. The present review summarizes the recent progress on the detection of UA by adopting electrochemical non- enzyme approaches. The electrochemical behavior of UA is introduced firstly, followed by a comprehensive review on the different types of materials used for electrode modification.

Chapter 2 - This review chapter examines the available evidence supporting the complex relationship between serum uric acid (sUA) and heart failure (HF).

Recently published literature indicates that hyperuricemia is a risk factor, as well as a risk marker for cardiovascular diseases. High sUA levels correlate with an increased risk of incident HF in community adults, and this incidence is related to hyperuricemia severity.

Hyperuricemia is common in established HF with reduced ejection fraction, with a higher prevalence in severely symptomatic patients. Elevated sUA levels are a prognostic marker, predicting adverse outcomes in terms of mortality and rehospitalization for acute HF and severe chronic systolic and diastolic HF. The responsible mechanisms for the deleterious effects of high uric acid levels in cardiovascular disease and the uric acid paradox will be briefly reviewed. The increased production of free oxygen radicals as a consequence of elevated xanthine-oxidase activity provides the basis for urate lowering therapy. Recent evidence and conflicting results related to urate lowering therapy with xanthine-oxidase inhibitors will also be summarized.

Chapter 3 - Acute decompensated heart failure (ADHF) is a family of related disorders, being defined as the new onset or recurrence of gradually or rapidly developing symptoms and signs of HF resulting in hospitalization and requiring urgent optimized therapy. ADHF has increasing incidence and poor prognosis, being a major cause for death and hospital readmission.

Hyperuricaemia is commonly found in patients with ADHF and has two main causes: an increase of the uric acid production because of higher abundance of purines and reduced renal function clearance, due to renal function impairment and/or diuretics treatment.

Most purines are metabolized by xanthine-oxidase (XO) particularly during hypoxia, acidosis and inflammation (present in ADHF). During this process, reactive oxygen species (ROS) are generated, leading to reduced nitric oxide release (with diminished endogenous vasodilatation and platelet aggregation) and increased oxidative stress, myocardial fibrosis, decreased cardiac muscle performance and reduced vascular tone.

Serum uric acid (sUA) may be a witness of XO upregulation, produced along with multiple ROS and may serve as a valuable biomarker for this activity in the cardiovascular system. In ADHF, the antioxidant activity of sUA demonstrated in some in-vitro studies is overcome by the pro-oxidant and pro-inflammatory effects of ROS accumulation (the sUA paradox). Hyperuricaemia was associated with greater degrees of pulmonary and systemic congestion, more vasoconstriction, and higher risk of death. Moreover, hyperuricaemia is associated with increased mortality, especially when it is a result of increased sUA production rather than decreased renal clearance.

The therapeutic approach of lowering UA levels and inhibiting XO activity can be an appealing strategy in HF. Previous studies showed that Allopurinol reduces sUA levels and myocardial oxygen consumption, improves endothelial function and reduces the serum concentration of BNP. In the authors' recent studies with Allopurinol, the authors saw a significant decrease of sUA levels and significant improvements of endothelial function.

SUA, this simple, inexpensive, widely available indicator, may serve as a valuable predictive biomarker, beyond traditional prognosis markers. Adding Allopurinol to the standard treatment can be a solution for improving endothelial function in ADHF, especially for patients with hyperuricaemia.

Chapter 4 - Allopurinol, a xanthine oxidase inhibitor, has significant evidence of beneficial effect in cardiovascular disease. However, there are conflicting data related to the efficacy of allopurinol treatment in arterial hypertension. The purpose of the study was the assessment of allopurinol effects on endothelial and platelet function in patients with controlled essential arterial hypertension.

Seventy six of one hundred thirty nine optimally treated hypertensive patients were randomly assigned to receive allopurinol 300 mg/day, regardless of serum uric acid level. Serum uric acid level, endothelial function (assessed by flow-mediated vasodilatation) and platelet aggregation response to adenosine diphosphate and collagen (by optical aggregometry method) were determined at baseline and after one month. Endothelial function was also reassessed after 3 and 6 months.

After allopurinol treatment, serum uric acid level significantly and persistently decreased, irrespective of the baseline level. In patients with allopurinol treatment blood pressure was slightly, but significantly lower. The endothelial function improved with allopurinol, more significantly in patients with higher cardiovascular risk. Allopurinol significantly decreased platelet aggregation to adenosine diphosphate and collagen, regardless of concomitant treatment with aspirin.

In conclusion, allopurinol could be an useful complementary treatment in arterial hypertension, having beneficial effects on endothelial and platelet function, essential pathogenic mechanisms in cardiovascular disease.

Chapter 5 - Tumor lysis syndrome is a rare, potentially life threatening condition that often occurs after chemotherapeutic treatment of various malignant neoplasms, especially high grade lymphomas. As the name implies, tumor lysis syndrome involves rapid tumor cell lysis which commonly results in elevated levels of uric acid and significant electrolyte imbalances. These abnormalities can result in crystal deposition in renal tubules and culminate in acute renal failure. An effective clinical management strategy is to preclude this condition by the administration of intravenous fluids and hypouricemic drugs. Historically, the drug of choice to treat tumor lysis syndrome has been allopurinol but in the last decade this has shifted to rasburicase. This recombinant urate oxidase efficiently converts uric acid to significantly more water soluble products thereby reducing the chances of acute renal failure. In 2002 this drug was approved for use in the United States by the Food and Drug Administration. Comparison studies have shown this treatment to be safer and more effective than allopurinol except for patients deficient in glucose-6-phosphate dehydrogenase where it is contraindicated. Patients treated with rasburicase need to have their uric acid levels vigilantly monitored and to ensure accuracy, the specimens should be kept on ice to minimize *ex vivo* breakdown.

Chapter 6 - Uric acid is one of the purine metabolites that animals have to excrete together with other nitrogen waste products such as ammonia and urea. Before being eliminated, uric acid circulates in blood and may precipitate as urate crystals when its concentration increases excessively, a situation known as “gout attack”. Besides its poor solubility, uric acid is a potent antioxidant in blood and should not be considered only as a potential toxic waste. Accordingly, uric acid levels change not only when nitrogen metabolism is altered but also during inflammatory, metabolic and cardiovascular diseases. Dietary polyphenols have been intensively studied in animal models of these diseases and reported to alleviate many of the complications of diabetes and obesity. The most known member of this family, resveratrol is now recognized for its antioxidant properties and for exhibiting promising beneficial effects, related to its cardioprotective, renoprotective, anti-inflammatory, antidiabetic and anti-obesity actions. However, the benefits of resveratrol are discussed regarding human health. In this context, the authors investigated the influence of a hydroxylated derivative of resveratrol, piceatannol, on obesity complications in an animal model exhibiting insulin resistance, dyslipidemia and early signs of nephropathy: the obese Zucker rat. The authors explored the changes in uric acid in conditions in which piceatannol reduced fibrosis biomarkers and lipid peroxidation in the kidney (repeated oral intake of 15 and 45 mg/kg/day for 6 weeks). Surprisingly, the renoprotective effect of piceatannol was not accompanied by a reduction of circulating uric acid, especially with the higher piceatannol dose, which increased by 30% the plasma uric acid. Both doses of piceatannol tended to decrease circulating triglycerides, and the higher dose decreased plasma non-esterified fatty acids and LDL-cholesterol while glycaemia and blood markers of glycation remained unaltered. Thus, in a situation indicating that piceatannol supplementation is improving lipid handling in obese rats, uric acid appeared to be negatively correlated with LDL-cholesterol levels and plasma triglycerides. Other analyses revealed that uric acid exhibited a positive relationship with kidney sirtuin (SIRT-1, related to antioxidant defences) and a negative relationship with kidney injury molecule (KIM-1, a marker that increases with renal dysfunction). In all, the authors' data indicated that an improvement of lipid handling could be induced by polyphenol supplementation without lowered uricemia. This suggested that moderately increased circulating uric acid could participate to delay renal dysfunctions, although severe hyperuricemia is deleterious since involved in kidney stone formation.

In: Uric Acid
Editor: Mary Newman

ISBN: 978-1-53610-287-1

Chapter 1

RECENT PROGRESS ON ELECTROCHEMICAL DETECTION OF URIC ACID

***Yuhong Zheng*[1*] *and Li Fu*[2]**
[1]Institute of Botany, Jiangsu Province and Chinese Academy of Sciences, Nanjing BotanicalGarden, Mem. Sun Yat-Sen, Nanjing, China
[2]Faculty of Science, Engineering and Technology, Swinburne University of Technology, Hawthorn, VIC, Australia

ABSTRACT

Uric acid (2,4,6-trihydroxypurine) (UA) is an end-product of purine derivatives in human metabolism. Excessive amount of it in serum is known as hyperuricemia and has been found to be related to hypertension, metabolic syndrome and cardiovascular disease. Therefore, fast and reliable detection of UA content in biological fluids is conventionally demanded for disease diagnosis and treatment. The present review summarizes the recent progress on the detection of UA by adopting electrochemical non- enzyme approaches. The electrochemical behavior of UA is introduced firstly, followed by a comprehensive review on the different types of materials used for electrode modification.

Keywords: uric acid, electrochemical determination, electrode modification, sensitivity, detection limit

[*]CorrespondingAuthorEmail:yuhongzhengcas@gmail.com.

INTRODUCTION

Uric acid (2,4,6-trihydroxypurine) (UA) is an end-product of purine derivatives in human metabolism [1]. Without further metabolism, it is excreted by kidneys and intestinal tract. Its serum concentration is controlled by the balance between production and excretion [2]. High concentration of UA in human body has been discovered to be associated with various diseases, such as gout, hyperuricaemia, Lesch-Nyan disease, obesity, diabetes, high cholesterol, hypertension, kidney disease and heart disease [3]. Hence monitoring the concentration of UA in biological fluids could give an early warning of these diseases and is indispensable for the diagnosis of several disorders. Various conditions may alter purine metabolism levels and make the UA to exceed the normal physiological ranges which should be 2×10^{-3}M in urine and $1.2–4.5\times10^{-4}$ M in blood. Since many of these abnormality occurred as a result of unhealthy diet and lifestyle, all patients with asymptomatic hyperuricemic should be encouraged to change their way of life, which necessitates working out an appropriate cost-effective monitoring system to provide adequate feedback and treatment guidelines to hyperuricemic patients.

The first method developed for uric acid analysis which is based on the chemical oxidation of uric acid to allantoin was introduced by Offer in 1894. It reduces phosphotungstic acid to a tungsten blue chromophoric compound. However, this method suffers several problems especially the interferences of the same reaction produced by other species [4]. A more substitutive approach is to use of uricase enzyme (UOX) so as to catalyze the uric acid oxidation to allantoin, H_2O_2 and CO_2.

Recently a considerable interest is aroused in the development of electrochemical sensors for UA detection, because the electrochemical sensors have some advantages of short analysis times, simple experimental procedures which can be applied to a variety of physiological samples, relatively cheaper instrumental requirements as well as high selectivity and sensitivity [5]. Though it is possible to measure the oxidation current of UA directly at common electrodes, it may result in overpotential, electrode fouling from oxidation products as well as an interference from some other biological molecules such as dopamine and ascorbic acid which undergo oxidation within the similar potential window as UA. Therefore, electrode surface modification was widely applied to enhance the analytical performance on the electrochemical detection of UA. The following section gives a comprehensive review on various materials recently used for non-enzyme electrode modification.

MATERIALS USED FOR ELECTRODE MODIFICATION

Carbon Based Nanomaterials

Due to its high electric conductivity, ability of analyte accumulating and surface fouling alleviation, as well as the capability to make surface functionalization and electrocatalysis activity, carbon might be the most widely used material in electroanalysis and electrocatalysis. It is chemically stable in most solution and can perform well in a wide range of temperatures. Carbon electrodes such as carbon paste and glassy carbon electrodes are commercially available and have the advantages of low cost, low background current and surface regeneration capability. In this section, we mainly focus on the application of carbon based nanomaterials as electrode surface modifier in UA sensors construction.

Since the first report on the electrochemical behavior of C_{60}in 1990, fullerene has been widely studied in the field of electrochemistry. It can lower the overpotential and enhance the electrochemical reaction rate. Therefore, it has been used as both redox catalysts and mediators in electrochemical sensor fabrication. Fullerene based electrochemical sensors have also been demonstrated for UA measurement with excellent performance [6].

Recent studies have indicated that carbon nanotube (CNT) can enhance the electrochemical reactivity of some electroactive biomolecules as well as promote their electron-transfer reactions. CNT-modified electrodes have also exhibited the capability of enhancing the sensibility of biomolecule accumulation on electrode.

Ardakani et al. [7] reported a modified carbon nanotube paste electrode by 2,2'-[1, 2-ethanediylbis(nitriloethylidyne)]-bis-hydroquinone. The prepared paste electrode showed a promising electrochemical performance towards the detection of UA. Zhang et al. [8]reported a novel functionalized SWCNT modified electrode and its application in determination of UA.

For MWCNT studies, Hu and co-workers reported a MWCNT-modified pyrolytic graphite electrode for determination of UA [9]. Similar reports were carried out by other research groups as well [10]. Surface modification was adopted to overcome the hydrophobicity of carbon materials. Reports showed that chitosan could be effectively used for MWCNT surface functionalization and consequently applied for UA sensor fabrication [11]. Besides MWCNT, MWCNT based composite materials have alsobeen widely used for electrode surface modification for UA measurement. For example, composites of lanthanum–MWCNT nanocomposites [12], graphene oxide-MWCNT nanocomposite [13], polyaniline-MWCNT composite film [14], congo red supported MWCNT [15], graphene–CNT [16], room temperature ionic liquid-MWCNT-chitosan [17], holmium fluoride nanoparticles-CNT [18], were investigated for uric acid sensing.

Carbon nanofibers (CNFs), having the similar mechanical strength and electric properties as CNTs and the diameter varying from some 10 to 500 nm, are also suitable to be used as electrocatalyst in electroanalysis. Recent electrochemical studies have shown that CNFs were capable of promoting the kinetics of electron transfer reaction. Yue et al. [19] demonstrated the preparation of a mesoporous carbon nanofiber-modified pyrolytic graphite electrode for UA detection. Using this method, anodic currents of UA is linear with their concentration in the range of 0.5–120 μM with detection limits of 0.2 μM. The good sensitivity and reproducibility of the proposed electrode make it be used as a good electrochemical sensor for the determination of UA in real sample analysis. Sun and co-workers demonstrated nitrogen-doped carbon nanofiber modified glassy carbon electrode for UA determination [20]. Nitrogen-doped carbon nanofiber modified GCE exhibited good electrocatalytic performance towards UA. The oxidation potentials were negatively shifted and the current responses were enhanced greatly compared with bare GCE.

Single-walled carbon nanohorn (SWCNH) is synthesized by laser ablation of pure graphite without using metal catalyst with high production rate and high yield. It is essentially metal-free and can be used directly for electrochemical and biosensing study. Typically, horn-shaped SWCNH assembles and forms dahlia-like or bud-like aggregates, ensuring extremely large surface area and fast mass transport. Due to its unique properties, SWCNH was applied for UA determination [21]. The oxidation overpotentials of UA decrease significantly and their oxidation peak currents increase dramatically at SWCNH-modified GCE.

Graphene has greatly attracted scientific and technological interest in recent years due to its large surface area, excellent thermal and electric conductivity and strong mechanical strength, which stand its unique physicochemical properties. It is the basic building block for graphitic materials of all other dimensionalities. Most graphene used in the fabrication of electrochemical sensor were produced through the reduction of grapheme oxide (GO).

Graphene has been directly used as electrode surface modifier. For example, Ping et al. [22] proposed an electrochemical UA sensor based on high-performance screen-printed graphene electrode, which showed excellent electrocatalytic activity for the oxidation of UA. Similar work was also carried out by other research groups [23].

Other graphene composites have been prepared include polymer functionalized graphene composites, noble metals incorporated graphene composites, metal oxide or hydroxide incorporated graphene composites and hemin functionalized graphene. For example, Liu and co-workers proposed a novel strategy based on overoxidized polyimidazole and graphene oxide (GO) copolymer modified electrode was proposed for the determination of UA [24]. Niu and co-workers reported a promising electrochemical sensor for determination of UA was fabricated based on the stacked graphene platelet nanofibers/ionic liquid/chitosan modified electrode [25]. Nancy and co-workers reported a novel solar graphene-nickel hydroxide modified glassy carbon electrode for UA determination [26]. The sensor exhibited appreciable electrocatalytic effect for the detection of lower concentrations of the analytes compared to solar graphene modified glassy carbon electrode.

Some metal oxides are good candidates for enhancing the electrochemical properties of electrodes. Therefore, several papers were focused on the development of graphene-metal oxides nanocomposites. For example, Fu and co-workers prepared reduced graphene oxide–ZnO nanorods composite via a simple one-pot hydrothermal approach. The synthesized reduced graphene oxide–ZnO nanorods composite has been successfully applied for GCE surface modification [27]. The reduced graphene oxide–ZnO nanorods composite-modified GCE was applied for sensitive and selective determination of UA. The biosensor exhibited a linear dependence on UA concentration ranging from 1 to 800 μM with a detection limit of 0.312 μM (S/N = 3). The proposed UA sensor also showed an excellent stability, reproducibility and anti-interference property.

In addition, element (or material) doped graphene has also been demonstrated to be able toenhance the electrochemical determination of AA (Ascorbic Acid). Sheng et al. [28] prepared nitrogen doped graphene via thermally annealing graphite oxide and melamine mixture. The electrochemical sensor based on nitrogen doped graphene was constructed to determination of UA. The electrochemical sensor shows a wide linear response for UA in the concentration range of 1.0×10^{-7} to 2.0×10^{-5} M with detection limit of 4.5×10^{-8} M at $S/N = 3$. Similar work with nitrogen doped graphene were studied by other research groups as well [29].

Composites made of twodifferent types of carbon nanomaterials were also favorable for electrochemical sensor fabrication. Du et al. [30a] coupled graphene flowers with carbon fibers for UA detection. Yang et al. [13] reported CTAB functionalized graphene oxide/multiwalled carbon nanotube composite modified electrode for UA detection. Du et al. [30b] fabricated a UA electrochemical sensor based on a carbon fiber electrode modified by layer-by-layer assembly of graphene and gold nanoparticles. Zhang and co-workers fabricated a graphene–carbon nanotube composite aerogel for selective detection of uric acid [16].

Other carbon based materials including mesoporous carbon [32], hollow nitrogen-doped carbon microspheres [33], porous carbon nanopolyhedra [34], were also synthesized and applied for the construction of uric acid electrochemical sensors.

Silica Based Materials

Mesoporous silica is one type of silica materials with distinctive properties, e.g., large surface area, tunable pore sizes and biocompatibility. It has attracted much attention and is broadly applied in catalysis, drug delivery, sorption and separation. For example, silica modified electrode could accumulate electro-active analytes onto electrode to enhance the current signal. In addition, silica can be grafted onto a variety of functional groups/materials to tune their surface properties. For example, Sun and co-workers demonstrated an electrochemical sensor using mesoporous SiO_2 as sensing material for the detection of UA [35]. With distinctive properties such as uniform porous networks, large surface area and high sorption ability, the mesoporous SiO_2 sensor exhibits remarkable surface enhancement effect, and greatly increases the response signals of UA. Gupta et al. [36] reported an Au NPs impregnated mesoporous silica spheres determination of UA.

Metal Hexacyanoferrates

Metal hexacyanoferrates are very interesting due to their electrochemical properties and have attracted considerable attention, as an excellent surface modifier, ever since their introduction in electrochemistry by Neff in 1978 via depositing a thin film of Prussian blue (PB) on an electrode surface [37]. Transition metal hexacyanoferrates belong to a class of important coordination complexes exhibiting several outstanding characteristics such as water insolubility, mixed valence, high ionic conductivity, and excellent redox mediator properties [38]. The electrode surfaces modification with metal hexacyanoferrate can be achieved via several routes including electrodeposition, adsorption and entrapping into a polymer matrix and mechanical attachment. Noroozifar et al. [39] reported a silver hexacyanoferrate nanoparticles/carbon nanotubes modified glassy carbon electrode for the determination of UA. Moreover, a cameroonian smectite clay has been transformed into Zn^{2+} homoionic form and then used to prepare film modified glassy carbon electrodes and carbon paste electrodes. These electrodes containing Zn^{2+} were exploited to prepare a mixed valence zinc hexacyanoferrate [40]. An interesting electrocatalytic properties toward UA were observed with these modified electrodes.

Conducting Electroactive Polymers

Discovered just two decades years ago, conductive polymers are originally proclaimed for their high conductivity/weight ratio. With their unique chemical and electronic properties, they are now arousing much attention. Most polymers are good candidates for surface modification because of their strong adherence to the electrode surface and stable in measurement.

Some reports showed electroactive polymer-coated electrode displayed excellent selectivity and sensitivity for the determination of UA. For example, a novel covalently modified GCE with poly (vinyl alcohol) has been fabricated through an electrochemical oxidation procedure and was used to electrochemically detect UA [41]. Yao et al. [42] reported a polymerized film of eriochrome black T (EBT) on the surface of a GCE in alkaline solution by cyclic voltammetry and subsequently for UA detection. Liu and co-workers demonstrated apoly (acrylic acid)- MWNTs composite-coated GCE for the determination of UA [43]. Other conductive electroactive polymers including poly (Evans Blue) [44],poly (acid chrome blue K) [45], poly (p-nitrobenzenazo resorcinol) [46], poly (sulfonazo III) [47], poly (N, N-dimethylaniline) [48], poly (n-butyl methacrylate) [49],poly (neutral red) [50], poly (calmagite) [51], Poly (p-aminobenzensulfonic acid) [52], poly (N-methylpyrrole) [53],Poly (4−vinylpyridine) [54], were investigated for uric acid sensing.

Among common conductive polymers, polyaniline has been widely studied and used in rechargeable batteries and electro-catalysis due to its high conductivity, good stability and redox reversibility. Several studies demonstrated the direct use of polyaniline for UA analysis [55]. However, polyaniline shows nearly no electroactivity when pH > 4. Chemical doping was used to overcome this problem and make it usable for biomolecules detection in neutral condition. For example, a composite film of polyaniline–poly (n-butyl methacrylate) composites were synthesized and applied for the electro-catalytic oxidation of UA [49]. Electrochemical synthesis of polyaniline nano-networks on p-aminobenzene sulfonic acid functionalized glassy carbon electrode is an alternative way for fabricating UA sensor [56]. Maivel et al. [57] prepared a Conducting polyaniline-graphene oxide fibrous nanocomposite for electrochemically determination of UA. Devi and Pundir reported a construction and application of an amperometric uric acid biosensor based on covalent immobilization of uricase on iron oxide nanoparticles/chitosan-g-polyaniline composite film electrodeposited on Pt electrode [58]. Polyaniline/Prussian blue composite can be electrochemically deposited on a platinum electrode for UA detection as well [59].

Metals

Noble metals (such as Au, Ag, Pt, Pd, Ru and their alloys) are excellent electrode materials due to their electro-conductivity and electrocatalytic properties. For Au nanostructures, Au-poly(luminol) hybrid film and MWCNT with incorporated β-cyclodextrin modified GCE was successfully prepared for determination of UA [60]. UA electrochemical sensor also can be established on a gold nanoparticle-decorated MoS_2[61]. Other reports using Au nanostructures for uric acid determination were also carried out [62]. Ag electrode possesses high conductivity and good stability in aqueous solution. In biosensor application, Ag ceramic graphite composite sensors have shown high performance for rapid, sensitive and selective determination of many biomolecules. Kaur et al. [63] reported the synthesis of silver nanoparticle-decorated reduced graphene oxide composite by heating the mixture of graphene oxide and silver nitrate aqueous solution in the presence of sodium hydroxide and used for fabricating electrochemical sensor for the determination of UA.

Many electrodes of pure metals exhibit unsatisfactory sensitivity, selectivity and are easy poisoned by adsorbed intermediates, which are critical issues for practical applications. Bimetallic systems were introduced for overcoming these disadvantages. For example, Chen and co-workers demonstrated the synthesis of bimetallic alloyed PdAg nanoflowers supported on reduced graphene oxide and subsequently used for electrode surface modification and detection of UA [64]. Liu et al. [65] fabricated an UA electrochemical sensor based on Au–Pt bimetallic nano-clusters. Murugavelu and co-workers studied the sensing ability of Ag–Pt nanoparticle are evaluated by opto and electrochemical method [66].

Table 1. Analytical performances of various modified electrodes for UA measurement

Detection methods	Electrode modifier	Linear detection range	Detection limr	Reference
DPV	Palladium nanoparticle-loaded carbon nanofibers	2-200μM	0.7 μM	[67]
DPV	MWNTs bridged mesocellular graphene foam nanocomposite	50 to 800μM	0.06 μM	[68]
DPV	2-amino-5-mercapto-[1,3,4] triazole self-assembled monolayers electrode	2.5 to 500 μM	0.08 μM	[69]
DPV	Exfoliated graphite paper electrode	0.5–35 μM	0.02 μM	[70]
CV	Meso-2,3-dimercaptosuccinic acid self-assembled gold electrode	0.8 to 5.0 mM	0.84 μM	[71]
DPV	L-cysteine self-assembled gold electrode	10 to 80 μM	2 μM	[72]
DPV	Co(TPP), tetraphenylborate Modified Glassy Carbon Electrode	0.1to 35 μM	0.06μM	[73]
DPV	1-butyl-4-methyl-pyridinium tetrafluroborate ionic liquid on carbon paste electrode	—	0.1 μM	[74]
DPV	Poly (tyrosine)/functionalized multi-walled carbon nanotubes composite film	0.1 to 350 μM	0.02 μM	[75]
DPV	Pristine graphene	6.00–1330 μM	4.82 μM	[76]
DPV	Hemin functionalized graphene oxide sheets	8 to 90 μM	0.5 μM	[77]
DPV	Helical carbon nanotubes	5.0–175 μM	0.08 μM	[78
DPV	Graphene anchored with Pd–Pt nanoparticles	4to 400μM	0.1 μM	[79]
DPV	Poly(l-arginine)/graphene composite film	0.1 to 10μM	0.1 μM	[80]
DPV	Reduced graphene oxide and Au nanoparticles entrapped in chitosan/silica sol–gel hybrid membranes	1.0–300 μM	0.6 μM	[81]
DPV	Electrochemically activated glassy carbon electrode	1to 55μM	0.07 μM	[82]
Ampero-metry	Ordered mesoporous carbon functionalized with ferrocenecarboxylic acid	60–390 μM	1.8 μM	[32] b
DPV	Choline and gold nanoparticles	1.2–100 μM	0.6 μM	[83]

Ionic Liquids

Room temperature ionic liquid is generally regarded as a compound which is entirely composed of organic cation and various inorganic anions which are in a liquid state under room temperature. Because it is with various physical and chemical properties such as wide electrochemical window, high ionic conductivity and good solubility, it will be more effectively enhance the electrochemical properties when adopting ionic liquid to do the modification of electrode than with bare electrodes. Zhao and co-workers studied the UA behavior at a GCE modified by a gel containing MWCNT and room-temperature ionic liquid of 1-octyl-3- methylimidazolium hexafluorophosphate [84]. Safavi and co-workers constructed carbon composite electrode using room temperature ionic liquid as pasting binder was employed as a novel electrode for sensitive determination of UA [85]. Rafati et al. [86] described the modification of a carbon paste electrode with MWCNT and an ionic liquid. Electrochemical studies revealed an optimized composition of 60% graphite, 20% paraffin, 10% MWCNT and 10% ionic liquid. In a next step, the optimized carbon paste electrode was modified with palladium nanoparticles by applying a double-pulse electrochemical technique. The resulting electrode showed excellent towards UA detection.

The analytical performances of some most illustrative modified electrodes in electrochemical determination of UA are summarized in Table 1.

CONCLUSION

Uric acid, as a primary end-product of purine metabolism, is contained in various body fluids. It is found that extremely abnormal UA content in body fluids is a symptom of some diseases. Therefore, simple and rapid method for UA detection in routine analysis is desirable. Based on oxidation of UA at bare electrodes, earlier electrochemical procedures suffered from varying degrees of interference from ascorbic acid which can be oxidized at a potential close to that of UA. This review summarized the recent development of chemically modified electrodes for electrochemical determination of UA. What's more, carbon based materials and conductive polymers were intensively studied as low-cost and high performance electrode surface modifiers for the fabrication of UA electrochemical sensors.

REFERENCES

[1] Grabowska, I.; Chudy, M.; Dybko, A.; Brzozka, Z., Uric acid determination in a miniaturized flow system with dual optical detection. *Sensors and Actuators B: Chemical* 2008,*130* (1), 508-513;(b) Kand'ár, R.; Žáková, P.; Mužáková, V., Monitoring of antioxidant properties of uric acid in humans for a consideration measuring of levels of allantoin in plasma by liquid chromatography. *Clinica Chimica Acta* 2006,*365* (1), 249-256.2.

[2] Dawson, J.; Walters, M., Uric acid and xanthine oxidase: future therapeutic targets in the prevention of cardiovascular disease? *British Journal of Clinical Pharmacology* 2006,*62* (6), 633-644.

[3] Alderman, M.; Aiyer, K. J., Uric acid: role in cardiovascular disease and effects of losartan. *Current medical research and opinion* 2004,*20* (3), 369-379; (b) Liberopoulos, E.; Christides, D.; Elisaf, M., Comparative effects of losartan and irbesartan on serum uric acid in hypertensive patients with hyperuricemia and gout. *Journal of Hypertension* 2002,*20* (2), 347; (c) Raj, C. R.; Ohsaka, T., Voltammetric detection of uric acid in the presence of ascorbic acid at a gold electrode modified with a self-assembled monolayer of heteroaromatic thiol. *Journal of Electroanalytical Chemistry* 2003,*540*, 69-77; (d) Huang, S.-H.; Shih, Y.-C.; Wu, C.-Y.; Yuan, C.-J.; Yang, Y.-S.; Li, Y.-K.; Wu, T.-K., Detection of serum uric acid using the optical polymeric enzyme biochip system. *Biosensors and Bioelectronics* 2004,*19* (12), 1627-1633; (e) Dutt, V. E.; Mottola, H., Determination of uric acid at the microgram level by a kinetic procedure based on a pseudo-induction period. *Anal. Chem.* 1974,*46* (12), 1777-1781; (f) Johnson, R. J.; Kang, D.-H.; Feig, D.; Kivlighn, S.; Kanellis, J.; Watanabe, S.; Tuttle, K. R.; Rodriguez-Iturbe, B.; Herrera-Acosta, J.; Mazzali, M., Is there a pathogenetic role for uric acid in hypertension and cardiovascular and renal disease? *Hypertension* 2003,*41* (6), 1183-1190.

[4] Galbán, J.; Andreu, Y.; Almenara, M.; de Marcos, S.; Castillo, J. R., Direct determination of uric acid in serum by a fluorometric-enzymatic method based on uricase. *Talanta* 2001,*54* (5), 847-854.

[5] Wring, S. A.; Hart, J. P., Chemically modified, carbon-based electrodes and their application as electrochemical sensors for the analysis of biologically important compounds. A review. *The Analyst* 1992,*117* (8), 1215-1229.

[6] Goyal, R. N.; Gupta, V. K.; Sangal, A.; Bachheti, N., Voltammetric Determination of Uric Acid at a Fullerene - C60 - Modified Glassy Carbon Electrode. *Electroanalysis* 2005,*17* (24), 2217-2223.

[7] Mazloum-Ardakani, M.; Beitollahi, H.; Ganjipour, B.; Naeimi, H.; Nejati, M., Electrochemical and catalytic investigations of dopamine and uric acid by modified carbon nanotube paste electrode. *Bioelectrochemistry* 2009,*75* (1), 1-8.

[8] Zhang, Y.; Pan, Y.; Su, S.; Zhang, L.; Li, S.; Shao, M., A Novel Functionalized Single - Wall Carbon Nanotube Modified Electrode and Its Application in Determination of Dopamine and Uric Acid in the Presence of High Concentrations of Ascorbic Acid. *Electroanalysis* 2007,*19* (16), 1695-1701.

[9] Liu, X.; Peng, Y.; Qu, X.; Ai, S.; Han, R.; Zhu, X., Multi-walled carbon nanotube-chitosanpoly (amidoamine)/DNA nanocomposite modified gold electrode for determination of dopamine and uric acid under coexistence of ascorbic acid. *Journal of Electroanalytical Chemistry* 2011,*654* (1–2), 72-78.

[10] Bi, H.; Li, Y.; Liu, S.; Guo, P.; Wei, Z.; Lv, C.; Zhang, J.; Zhao, X., Carbon-nanotube-modified glassy carbon electrode for simultaneous determination of dopamine, ascorbic acid and uric acid: The effect of functional groups. *Sensors and Actuators B: Chemical* 2012,*171*, 1132-1140;(b) Alwarappan, S.; Liu, G.; Li, C.-Z., Simultaneous detection of dopamine, ascorbic acid, and uric acid at electrochemically pretreated carbon nanotube biosensors. *Nanomedicine: Nanotechnology, Biology and Medicine* 2010,*6* (1), 52-57;(c) Sun, Y.-Y.; Wu, K.-B.; Hu, S.-S., Selective determination of dopamine in the presence of high concentration ascorbic acid and uric acid using carbon nanotube modified glassy carbon electrode. *Chemical Journal of Chinese Universities-Chinese edition* 2002,*23* (11), 2067-2069;(d) Thomas, T.; Mascarenhas, R. J.; Martis, P.; Mekhalif, Z.; Swamy, B. K., Multi-walled carbon nanotube modified carbon paste electrode as an electrochemical sensor for the determination of epinephrine in the presence of ascorbic acid and uric acid. *Materials Science and Engineering: C* 2013,*33* (6), 3294-3302.

[11] Lu, G.; Jiang, L.; Song, F.; Liu, C.; Jiang, L., Determination of Uric Acid and Norepinephrine by Chitosan - Multiwall Carbon Nanotube Modified Electrode. *Electroanalysis* 2005,*17* (10), 901-905.

[12] Zhang, W.; Yuan, R.; Chai, Y.-Q.; Zhang, Y.; Chen, S.-H., A simple strategy based on lanthanum–multiwalled carbon nanotube nanocomposites for simultaneous determination of ascorbic acid, dopamine, uric acid and nitrite. *Sensors and Actuators B: Chemical* 2012,*166*, 601-607.

[13] Yang, Y. J.; Li, W., CTAB functionalized graphene oxide/multiwalled carbon nanotube composite modified electrode for the simultaneous determination of ascorbic acid, dopamine, uric acid and nitrite. *Biosensors and Bioelectronics* 2014,*56*, 300-306.

[14] Bhambi, M.; Sumana, G.; Malhotra, B.; Pundir, C., An amperomertic uric acid biosensor based on immobilization of uricase onto polyaniline-multiwalled carbon nanotube composite film. *Artificial Cells, Blood Substitutes, and Biotechnology* 2010,*38* (4), 178-185.

[15] Shahrokhian, S.; Zare-Mehrjardi, H. R.; Khajehsharifi, H., Modification of carbon paste with congo red supported on multi-walled carbon nanotube for voltammetric determination of uric acid in the presence of ascorbic acid. *Journal of Solid State Electrochemistry* 2009,*13* (10), 1567-1575.

[16] Zhang, F.; Tang, J.; Wang, Z.; Qin, L.-C., Graphene–carbon nanotube composite aerogel for selective detection of uric acid. *Chemical Physics Letters* 2013,*590*, 121-125.

[17] Kianipour, S.; Asghari, A., Room temperature ionic liquid/multiwalled carbon nanotube/chitosan-modified glassy carbon electrode as a sensor for simultaneous determination of ascorbic acid, uric acid, acetaminophen, and mefenamic acid. *IEEE Sensors Journal* 2013,*13* (7), 2690-2698.

[18] Noroozifar, M.; Khorasani-Motlagh, M.; Jahromi, F. Z.; Rostami, S., Sensitive and selective determination of uric acid in real samples by modified glassy carbon electrode with holmium fluoride nanoparticles/multi-walled carbon nanotube as a new biosensor. *Sensors and Actuators B: Chemical* 2013,*188*, 65-72.

[19] Yue, Y.; Hu, G.; Zheng, M.; Guo, Y.; Cao, J.; Shao, S., A mesoporous carbon nanofiber-modified pyrolytic graphite electrode used for the simultaneous determination of dopamine, uric acid, and ascorbic acid. *Carbon* 2012,*50* (1), 107-114.

[20] Sun, J.; Li, L.; Zhang, X.; Liu, D.; Lv, S.; Zhu, D.; Wu, T.; You, T., Simultaneous determination of ascorbic acid, dopamine and uric acid at a nitrogen-doped carbon nanofiber modified electrode. *RSC Advances* 2015,*5* (16), 11925-11932.

[21] Zhu, S.; Li, H.; Niu, W.; Xu, G., Simultaneous electrochemical determination of uric acid, dopamine, and ascorbic acid at single-walled carbon nanohorn modified glassy carbon electrode. *Biosensors and Bioelectronics* 2009,*25* (4), 940-943.

[22] Ping, J.; Wu, J.; Wang, Y.; Ying, Y., Simultaneous determination of ascorbic acid, dopamine and uric acid using high-performance screen-printed graphene electrode. *Biosensors and Bioelectronics* 2012,*34* (1), 70-76.

[23] Mallesha, M.; Manjunatha, R.; Nethravathi, C.; Suresh, G. S.; Rajamathi, M.; Melo, J. S.; Venkatesha, T. V., Functionalized-graphene modified graphite electrode for the selective determination of dopamine in presence of uric acid and ascorbic acid. *Bioelectrochemistry* 2011,*81* (2), 104-108;(b) Lian, Q.; He, Z.; He, Q.; Luo, A.; Yan, K.; Zhang, D.; Lu, X.; Zhou, X., Simultaneous determination of ascorbic acid, dopamine and uric acid based on tryptophan functionalized graphene. *Anal. Chim. Acta.* 2014,*823*, 32-39;(c) Raj, M. A.; John, S. A., Simultaneous determination of uric acid, xanthine, hypoxanthine and caffeine in human blood serum and urine samples using electrochemically reduced graphene oxide modified electrode. *Anal. Chim. Acta.* 2013,*771*, 14-20.

[24] Liu, X.; Zhang, L.; Wei, S.; Chen, S.; Ou, X.; Lu, Q., Overoxidized polyimidazole/graphene oxide copolymer modified electrode for the simultaneous determination of ascorbic acid, dopamine, uric acid, guanine and adenine. *Biosensors and Bioelectronics* 2014,*57*, 232-238.

[25] Niu, X.; Yang, W.; Guo, H.; Ren, J.; Yang, F.; Gao, J., A novel and simple strategy for simultaneous determination of dopamine, uric acid and ascorbic acid based on the stacked graphene platelet nanofibers/ionic liquids/chitosan modified electrode. *Talanta* 2012,*99*, 984-988.

[26] Nancy, T. E. M.; Kumary, V. A., Synergistic electrocatalytic effect of graphene/nickel hydroxide composite for the simultaneous electrochemical determination of ascorbic acid, dopamine and uric acid. *Electrochimica Acta* 2014,*133*, 233-240.

[27] Fu, L.; Zheng, Y.; Wang, A.; Cai, W.; Deng, B.; Zhang, Z., An electrochemical sensor based on reduced graphene oxide and ZnO nanorods-modified glassy carbon electrode for uric acid detection. *Arab J Sci Eng* 2016,*41* (1), 135-141.

[28] Sheng, Z.-H.; Zheng, X.-Q.; Xu, J.-Y.; Bao, W.-J.; Wang, F.-B.; Xia, X.-H., Electrochemical sensor based on nitrogen doped graphene: Simultaneous determination of ascorbic acid, dopamine and uric acid. *Biosensors and Bioelectronics* 2012,*34* (1), 125-131.

[29] LI, N.-B.; HE, F.-Y.; Li, L.; HU, Y.-J.; BAI, C.-C.; DUAN, Y.-Q., Selective Determination of Uric Acid at Nitrogen-doped Graphene/Chitosan Composite Modified Electrode in the Presence of a Large Amount of Ascorbic Acid. *Chinese Journal of Analytical Chemistry* 2015,*12*, 013;(b) Biswas, S.; Das, R.; Chakraborty, D.; Bandhyopadhyay, R.; Pramanik, P., Synthesis of Nitrogen Doped Multilayered Graphene Flakes: Selective Non - enzymatic Electrochemical Determination of Dopamine and Uric Acid in presence of Ascorbic Acid. *Electroanalysis* 2015,*27* (5), 1253-1261;(c) Luo, A.; Lian, Q.; An, Z.; Li, Z.; Guo, Y.; Zhang, D.; Xue, Z.; Zhou, X.; Lu, X., Simultaneous determination of uric acid, xanthine and hypoxanthine based on sulfonic groups functionalized nitrogen-doped graphene. *Journal of Electroanalytical Chemistry* 2015,*756*, 22-29;(d) Li, S.-M.; Yang, S.-Y.; Wang, Y.-S.; Lien, C.-H.; Tien, H.-W.; Hsiao, S.-T.; Liao, W.-H.; Tsai, H.-P.; Chang, C.-L.; Ma, C.-C. M., Controllable synthesis of nitrogen-doped graphene and its effect on the simultaneous electrochemical determination of ascorbic acid, dopamine, and uric acid. *Carbon* 2013,*59*, 418-429.

[30] Du, J.; Yue, R.; Ren, F.; Yao, Z.; Jiang, F.; Yang, P.; Du, Y., Novel graphene flowers modified carbon fibers for simultaneous determination of ascorbic acid, dopamine and uric acid. *Biosensors and Bioelectronics* 2014,*53*, 220-224.

[31] Du, J.; Yue, R.; Ren, F.; Yao, Z.; Jiang, F.; Yang, P.; Du, Y., Simultaneous determination of uric acid and dopamine using a carbon fiber electrode modified by layer-by-layer assembly of graphene and gold nanoparticles. *Gold Bull* 2013,*46* (3), 137-144.

[32] Zheng, D.; Ye, J.; Zhou, L.; Zhang, Y.; Yu, C., Simultaneous determination of dopamine, ascorbic acid and uric acid on ordered mesoporous carbon/Nafion composite film. *Journal of Electroanalytical Chemistry* 2009,*625* (1), 82-87;(b) Ndamanisha, J. C.; Guo, L., Electrochemical determination of uric acid at ordered mesoporous carbon functionalized with ferrocenecarboxylic acid-modified electrode. *Biosensors and Bioelectronics* 2008,*23* (11), 1680-1685.

[33] Xiao, C.; Chu, X.; Yang, Y.; Li, X.; Zhang, X.; Chen, J., Hollow nitrogen-doped carbon microspheres pyrolyzed from self-polymerized dopamine and its application in simultaneous electrochemical determination of uric acid, ascorbic acid and dopamine. *Biosensors and Bioelectronics* 2011,*26* (6), 2934-2939.

[34] Gai, P.; Zhang, H.; Zhang, Y.; Liu, W.; Zhu, G.; Zhang, X.; Chen, J., Simultaneous electrochemical detection of ascorbic acid, dopamine and uric acid based on nitrogen doped porous carbon nanopolyhedra. *Journal of Materials Chemistry B* 2013,*1* (21), 2742-2749.

[35] Sun, D.; Zhang, Y.; Wang, F.; Wu, K.; Chen, J.; Zhou, Y., Electrochemical sensor for simultaneous detection of ascorbic acid, uric acid and xanthine based on the surface enhancement effect of mesoporous silica. *Sensors and Actuators B: Chemical* 2009,*141* (2), 641-645.

[36] Gupta, R.; Ganesan, V., Gold nanoparticles impregnated mesoporous silica spheres for simultaneous and selective determination of uric acid and ascorbic acid. *Sensors and Actuators B: Chemical* 2015,*219*, 139-145.

[37] Neff, V. D., Electrochemical oxidation and reduction of thin films of Prussian Blue. *Journal of the Electrochemical Society* 1978,*125* (6), 886-887.

[38] Sinha, S.; Humphrey, B. D.; Bocarsly, A. B., Reaction of nickel electrode surfaces with anionic metal-cyanide complexes: formation of precipitated surfaces. *Inorganic Chemistry* 1984,*23* (2), 203-212;(b) Kulesza, P. J.; Galus, Z., Mixed-valence electron hopping, redox conduction and migration effects in solid-state electrochemistry of transition metal hexacyanoferrates. *Journal of Electroanalytical Chemistry* 1992,*323* (1), 261-274;(c) Yang, M.; Jiang, J.; Yang, Y.; Chen, X.; Shen, G.; Yu, R., Carbon nanotube/cobalt hexacyanoferrate nanoparticle-biopolymer system for the fabrication of biosensors. *Biosensors and Bioelectronics* 2006,*21* (9), 1791-1797.

[39] Noroozifar, M.; Khorasani-Motlagh, M.; Taheri, A., Preparation of silver hexacyanoferrate nanoparticles and its application for the simultaneous determination of ascorbic acid, dopamine and uric acid. *Talanta* 2010,*80* (5), 1657-1664.

[40] Kemmegne ‐ Mbouguen, J. C.; Angnes, L.; Mouafo ‐ Tchinda, E.; Ngameni, E., Electrochemical Determination of Uric Acid, Dopamine and Tryptophan at Zinc Hexacyanoferrate Clay Modified Electrode. *Electroanalysis* 2015,*27* (10), 2387-2398.

[41] Li, Y.; Lin, X., Simultaneous electroanalysis of dopamine, ascorbic acid and uric acid by poly (vinyl alcohol) covalently modified glassy carbon electrode. *Sensors and Actuators B: Chemical* 2006,*115* (1), 134-139.

[42] Yao, H.; Sun, Y.; Lin, X.; Tang, Y.; Huang, L., Electrochemical characterization of poly(eriochrome black T) modified glassy carbon electrode and its application to simultaneous determination of dopamine, ascorbic acid and uric acid. *Electrochimica Acta* 2007,*52* (20), 6165-6171.

[43] Liu, A.; Honma, I.; Zhou, H., Simultaneous voltammetric detection of dopamine and uric acid at their physiological level in the presence of ascorbic acid using poly(acrylic acid)-multiwalled carbon-nanotube composite-covered glassy-carbon electrode. *Biosensors and Bioelectronics* 2007,*23* (1), 74-80.

[44] Lin, L.; Chen, J.; Yao, H.; Chen, Y.; Zheng, Y.; Lin, X., Simultaneous determination of dopamine, ascorbic acid and uric acid at poly (Evans Blue) modified glassy carbon electrode. *Bioelectrochemistry* 2008,*73* (1), 11-17.

[45] Zhang, R.; Jin, G.-D.; Chen, D.; Hu, X.-Y., Simultaneous electrochemical determination of dopamine, ascorbic acid and uric acid using poly (acid chrome blue K) modified glassy carbon electrode. *Sensors and Actuators B: Chemical* 2009,*138* (1), 174-181.

[46] Lin, X.; Zhang, Y.; Chen, W.; Wu, P., Electrocatalytic oxidation and determination of dopamine in the presence of ascorbic acid and uric acid at a poly (p-nitrobenzenazo resorcinol) modified glassy carbon electrode. *Sensors and Actuators B: Chemical* 2007,*122* (1), 309-314.

[47] Ensafi, A. A.; Taei, M.; Khayamian, T.; Arabzadeh, A., Highly selective determination of ascorbic acid, dopamine, and uric acid by differential pulse voltammetry using poly (sulfonazo III) modified glassy carbon electrode. *Sensors and Actuators B: Chemical* 2010,*147* (1), 213-221.

[48] Roy, P. R.; Okajima, T.; Ohsaka, T., Simultaneous electrochemical detection of uric acid and ascorbic acid at a poly (N, N-dimethylaniline) film-coated GC electrode. *Journal of electroanalytical chemistry* 2004,*561*, 75-82.

[49] Castillo-Ortega, M.; Rodriguez, D.; Encinas, J.; Plascencia, M.; Mendez-Velarde, F.; Olayo, R., Conductometric uric acid and urea biosensor prepared from electroconductive polyaniline–poly (n-butyl methacrylate) composites. *Sensors and Actuators B: Chemical* 2002,*85* (1), 19-25.

[50] Yogeswaran, U.; Chen, S.-M., Separation and concentration effect of f-MWCNTs on electrocatalytic responses of ascorbic acid, dopamine and uric acid at f-MWCNTs incorporated with poly (neutral red) composite films. *Electrochimica Acta* 2007,*52* (19), 5985-5996.

[51] Chandra, U.; Swamy, B. K.; Gilbert, O.; Sherigara, B., Voltammetric resolution of dopamine in the presence of ascorbic acid and uric acid at poly (calmagite) film coated carbon paste electrode. *Electrochimica Acta* 2010,*55* (24), 7166-7174.

[52] Lin, X.; Kang, G.; Lu, L., DNA/Poly (p-aminobenzensulfonic acid) composite bi-layer modified glassy carbon electrode for determination of dopamine and uric acid under coexistence of ascorbic acid. *Bioelectrochemistry* 2007,*70* (2), 235-244.

[53] Atta, N. F.; El-Kady, M. F.; Galal, A., Simultaneous determination of catecholamines, uric acid and ascorbic acid at physiological levels using poly (N-methylpyrrole)/Pd-nanoclusters sensor. *Analytical Biochemistry* 2010,*400* (1), 78-88.

[54] Zen, J. M.; Chen, Y. J.; Hsu, C. T.; Ting, Y. S., Poly (4 - vinylpyridine) - coated chemically modified electrode for the detection of uric acid in the presence of a high concentration of ascorbic acid. *Electroanalysis* 1997,*9* (13), 1009-1013.

[55] Prathap, M. A.; Srivastava, R., Tailoring properties of polyaniline for simultaneous determination of a quaternary mixture of ascorbic acid, dopamine, uric acid, and tryptophan. *Sensors and Actuators B: Chemical* 2013,*177*, 239-250;(b) Guiping, H.; Ping, Z., Determination of Uric Acid by Differential Pulse Voltammetry with Glassy Carbon Electrode Modified by Polyaniline. *Chemical Analysis and Meterage* 2006,*15* (1), 33;(c) Liang, R.; He, C.X., Electro-separation of dopamine, uric acid and ascorbic acid based on a graphite electrode modified polyaniline. *Journal of Science of Teachers' College and University* 2011,*1*, 028.

[56] Zhang, L.; Zhang, C.; Lian, J., Electrochemical synthesis of polyaniline nano-networks on p-aminobenzene sulfonic acid functionalized glassy carbon electrode: Its use for the simultaneous determination of ascorbic acid and uric acid. *Biosensors and Bioelectronics* 2008,*24* (4), 690-695.

[57] Manivel, P.; Dhakshnamoorthy, M.; Balamurugan, A.; Ponpandian, N.; Mangalaraj, D.; Viswanathan, C., Conducting polyaniline-graphene oxide fibrous nanocomposites: preparation, characterization and simultaneous electrochemical detection of ascorbic acid, dopamine and uric acid. *Rsc Advances* 2013,*3* (34), 14428-14437.

[58] Devi, R.; Pundir, C. S., Construction and application of an amperometric uric acid biosensor based on covalent immobilization of uricase on iron oxide nanoparticles/chitosan-g-polyaniline composite film electrodeposited on Pt electrode. *Sensors and Actuators B: Chemical* 2014,*193*, 608-615.

[59] Thakur, B.; Sawant, S. N., Polyaniline/Prussian - Blue - Based Amperometric Biosensor for Detection of Uric Acid. *ChemPlusChem* 2013,*78* (2), 166-174.

[60] Jia, D.; Dai, J.; Yuan, H.; Lei, L.; Xiao, D., Selective detection of dopamine in the presence of uric acid using a gold nanoparticles-poly(luminol) hybrid film and multi-walled carbon nanotubes with incorporated β-cyclodextrin modified glassy carbon electrode. *Talanta* 2011,*85* (5), 2344-2351.

[61] Sun, H.; Chao, J.; Zuo, X.; Su, S.; Liu, X.; Yuwen, L.; Fan, C.; Wang, L., Gold nanoparticle-decorated MoS2 nanosheets for simultaneous detection of ascorbic acid, dopamine and uric acid. *RSC Advances* 2014,*4* (52), 27625-27629.

[62] Huang, X.; Lan, T.; Zhang, B.; Ren, J., Gold nanoparticle–enzyme conjugates based FRET for highly sensitive determination of hydrogen peroxide, glucose and uric acid using tyramide reaction. *The Analyst* 2012,*137* (16), 3659-3666;(b) Zhang, W.; Chai, Y.; Yuan, R.; Han, J.; Chen, S., Deposited gold nanocrystals enhanced porous PTCA–Cys layer for simultaneous detection of ascorbic acid, dopamine and uric acid. *Sensors and Actuators B: Chemical* 2013,*183*, 157-162;(c) Ahuja, T.; Tanwar, V.; Mishra, S.; Kumar, D.; Biradar, A., Immobilization of uricase enzyme on self-assembled gold nanoparticles for application in uric acid biosensor. *Journal of Nanoscience and Nanotechnology* 2011,*11* (6), 4692-4701;(d) Wang, J.; Zhang, W.-D., Sputtering deposition of gold nanoparticles onto vertically aligned carbon nanotubes for electroanalysis of uric acid. *Journal of electroanalytical chemistry* 2011,*654* (1), 79-84;(e) Dorraji, P. S.; Jalali, F., Novel sensitive electrochemical sensor for simultaneous determination of epinephrine and uric acid by using a nanocomposite of MWCNTs–chitosan and gold nanoparticles attached to thioglycolic acid. *Sensors and Actuators B: Chemical* 2014,*200*, 251-258;(f) Benvidi, A.; Dehghani-Firouzabadi, A.; Mazloum-Ardakani, M.; Mirjalili, B.-B. F.; Zare, R., Electrochemical deposition of gold nanoparticles on reduced graphene oxide modified glassy carbon electrode for simultaneous

determination of levodopa, uric acid and folic acid. *Journal of Electroanalytical Chemistry* 2015,*736*, 22-29.

[63] Kaur, B.; Pandiyan, T.; Satpati, B.; Srivastava, R., Simultaneous and sensitive determination of ascorbic acid, dopamine, uric acid, and tryptophan with silver nanoparticles-decorated reduced graphene oxide modified electrode. *Colloids and Surfaces B: Biointerfaces* 2013,*111*, 97-106.

[64] Chen, L.-X.; Zheng, J.-N.; Wang, A.-J.; Wu, L.-J.; Chen, J.-R.; Feng, J.-J., Facile synthesis of porous bimetallic alloyed PdAg nanoflowers supported on reduced graphene oxide for simultaneous detection of ascorbic acid, dopamine, and uric acid. *The Analyst* 2015,*140* (9), 3183-3192.

[65] Liu, Y.; She, P.; Gong, J.; Wu, W.; Xu, S.; Li, J.; Zhao, K.; Deng, A., A novel sensor based on electrodeposited Au–Pt bimetallic nano-clusters decorated on graphene oxide (GO)–electrochemically reduced GO for sensitive detection of dopamine and uric acid. *Sensors and Actuators B: Chemical* 2015,*221*, 1542-1553.

[66] Murugavelu, M.; Loganathan, B.; Karthikeyan, B., Opto and Electrochemical Sensing of Uric Acid with Bimetallic Nano Ag–Pt Particles. *Sensor Letters* 2013,*11* (4), 632-635.

[67] Huang, J.; Liu, Y.; Hou, H.; You, T., Simultaneous electrochemical determination of dopamine, uric acid and ascorbic acid using palladium nanoparticle-loaded carbon nanofibers modified electrode. *Biosensors and Bioelectronics* 2008,*24* (4), 632-637.

[68] Li, H.; Wang, Y.; Ye, D.; Luo, J.; Su, B.; Zhang, S.; Kong, J., An electrochemical sensor for simultaneous determination of ascorbic acid, dopamine, uric acid and tryptophan based on MWNTs bridged mesocellular graphene foam nanocomposite. *Talanta* 2014,*127*, 255-261.

[69] Liu, C.; Lu, G.; Jiang, L.; Jiang, L.; Zhou, X., Study on the Electrochemical Behavior of Dopamine and Uric Acid at a 2 - Amino - 5 - mercapto - [1, 3, 4] Triazole Self - Assembled Monolayers Electrode. *Electroanalysis* 2006,*18* (3), 291-297.

[70] Cai, W.; Lai, T.; Du, H.; Ye, J., Electrochemical determination of ascorbic acid, dopamine and uric acid based on an exfoliated graphite paper electrode: A high performance flexible sensor. *Sensors and Actuators B: Chemical* 2014,*193*, 492-500.

[71] Li, N. B.; Niu, L. M.; Luo, H. Q., Electrochemical behavior of uric acid and epinephrine at a meso-2, 3-dimercaptosuccinic acid self-assembled gold electrode. *Microchim. Acta.* 2006,*153* (1-2), 37-44.

[72] Ical, E., Simultaneous electrochemical determination of uric acid and ascorbic acid using L-cysteine self-assembled gold electrode. *Int. J. Electrochem. Sci* 2006,*1*, 363-371.

[73] Zeng, Y.; Li, C.; Tang, C.; Zhang, X. B.; Shen, G.; Yu, R., The electrochemical properties of Co (TPP), tetraphenylborate modified glassy carbon electrode: application to dopamine and uric acid analysis. *Electroanalysis* 2006,*18* (5), 440-448.

[74] Pandurangachar, M.; Swamy, B. E. K.; Chandrashekar, B. N.; Gilbert, O.; Sherigara, B. S., Electrochemical deposition of 1-butyl-4-methyl-pyridinium tetrafluroborate ionic liquid on carbon paste electrode and its application for the simultaneous determination of dopamine, ascorbic acid and uric acid. *Journal of Molecular Liquids* 2011,*158* (1), 13-17.

[75] Wang, Y.; Bi, C., Simultaneous electrochemical determination of ascorbic acid, dopamine and uric acid using poly (tyrosine)/ functionalized multi-walled carbon nanotubes composite film modified electrode. *Journal of Molecular Liquids* 2013,*177*, 26-31.

[76] Qi, S.; Zhao, B.; Tang, H.; Jiang, X., Determination of ascorbic acid, dopamine, and uric acid by a novel electrochemical sensor based on pristine graphene. *Electrochimica Acta* 2015,*161*, 395-402.

[77] Zou, H. L.; Li, B. L.; Luo, H. Q.; Li, N. B., A novel electrochemical biosensor based on hemin functionalized graphene oxide sheets for simultaneous determination of ascorbic acid, dopamine and uric acid. *Sensors and Actuators B: Chemical* 2015,*207, Part A*, 535-541.

[78] Zhang, B.; Huang, D.; Xu, X.; Alemu, G.; Zhang, Y.; Zhan, F.; Shen, Y.; Wang, M., Simultaneous electrochemical determination of ascorbic acid, dopamine and uric acid with helical carbon nanotubes. *Electrochimica Acta* 2013,*91*, 261-266.

[79] Yan, J.; Liu, S.; Zhang, Z.; He, G.; Zhou, P.; Liang, H.; Tian, L.; Zhou, X.; Jiang, H., Simultaneous electrochemical detection of ascorbic acid, dopamine and uric acid based on graphene anchored with Pd–Pt nanoparticles. *Colloids and Surfaces B: Biointerfaces* 2013,*111*, 392-397.

[80] Zhang, F.; Wang, Z.; Zhang, Y.; Zheng, Z.; Wang, C.; Du, Y.; Ye, W., Simultaneous electrochemical determination of uric acid, xanthine and hypoxanthine based on poly(l-arginine)/graphene composite film modified electrode. *Talanta* 2012,*93*, 320-325.

[81] Liu, X.; Xie, L.; Li, H., Electrochemical biosensor based on reduced graphene oxide and Au nanoparticles entrapped in chitosan/silica sol–gel hybrid membranes for determination of dopamine and uric acid. *Journal of Electroanalytical Chemistry* 2012,*682*, 158-163.

[82] Qiao, J. X.; Luo, H. Q.; Li, N. B., Electrochemical behavior of uric acid and epinephrine at an electrochemically activated glassy carbon electrode. *Colloids and Surfaces B: Biointerfaces* 2008,*62* (1), 31-35.

[83] Wang, P.; Li, Y.; Huang, X.; Wang, L., Fabrication of layer-by-layer modified multilayer films containing choline and gold nanoparticles and its sensing application for electrochemical determination of dopamine and uric acid. *Talanta* 2007,*73* (3), 431-437.

[84] Zhao, Y.; Gao, Y.; Zhan, D.; Liu, H.; Zhao, Q.; Kou, Y.; Shao, Y.; Li, M.; Zhuang, Q.; Zhu, Z., Selective detection of dopamine in the presence of ascorbic acid and uric acid by a carbon nanotubes-ionic liquid gel modified electrode. *Talanta* 2005,*66* (1), 51-57.

[85] Safavi, A.; Maleki, N.; Moradlou, O.; Tajabadi, F., Simultaneous determination of dopamine, ascorbic acid, and uric acid using carbon ionic liquid electrode. *Analytical Biochemistry* 2006,*359* (2), 224-229.

[86] Rafati, A. A.; Afraz, A.; Hajian, A.; Assari, P., Simultaneous determination of ascorbic acid, dopamine, and uric acid using a carbon paste electrode modified with multiwalled carbon nanotubes, ionic liquid, and palladium nanoparticles. *Microchim. Acta.* 2014,*181* (15-16), 1999-2008.

BIOGRAPHICAL SKETCH

Yuhong Zheng

Affiliation: Institute of Botany, Jiangsu Province and Chinese Academy of Sciences, Nanjing Botanical Garden, Mem. Sun Yat-Sen, Nanjing 210014, China

Education:

09/2001-12/2006 Ph.D. (Phytology), College of Life Sciences, Nanjing Agricultural University, Nanjing, Specialization in Plant Plant Systematic and phylogeny; Thesis topic: Study on Systematic Biology of Sect. *Enantiophyllum* in *Dioscorea* L. in China.

09/1998-07/2001 Master (Phytology), Institute of Botany and Jiangsu Province and Chinese Academy of Sciences, Jiangsu, Specialization in Plant physiology; Thesis topic: A study on low temperature hardiness of germplasm resources of *Cynodon dactylon* (L.) Pers. in China.

09/1993-07/1995Biology Education, Department of Biology, Zhoukou Normal College, Henan.

Research and Professional Experience:

12/2006-Present: Institute of Botany, Jiangsu Province and Chinese Academy of Sciences, Nanjing Botanical Garden, Mem. Sun Yat-Sen

Professional Appointments:

12/2006-09/2011: Assistant Professor,Institute of Botany, Jiangsu Province and Chinese Academy of Sciences, Nanjing Botanical Garden, Mem. Sun Yat-Sen

10/2011-Present: Associated Professor, Institute of Botany, Jiangsu Province and Chinese Academy of Sciences, Nanjing Botanical Garden, Mem. Sun Yat-Sen

Publications Last 3 Years:

Aiwu Wang, Hoi Pong Ng, Yi Xu, Yuyu Li, Yuhong Zheng*, Jinping Yu, Fugui Han, Feng Peng and Li Fu. Gold Nanoparticles: Synthesis, Stability Test, and Application for the Rice Growth[J]. Journal of Nanomaterials, 2014, http://dx.doi.org/10.1155 /2014 /451232.

Li Fu, Yuhong Zheng*, Quanjin Ren, Aiwu Wang, Bo Deng. Green Biosynthesis of SnO_2 Nanoparticles by *Plectranthus amboinicus* Leaf Extract Their Photocatalytic Activity Toward Rhodamine B Degradation [J]. Journal of Ovonic Research, 2015, 11(1): 21-26.

In: Uric Acid
Editor: Mary Newman

ISBN: 978-1-53610-287-1

Chapter 2

URIC ACID AND HEART FAILURE

Adriana Ilieşiu**, *MD, PhD, FESC

Department of Internal Medicine and Cardiology, "Carol Davila" University of Medicine and Pharmacy, "Theodor Burghele" Clinical Hospital, Bucharest, Romania

ABSTRACT

This review chapter examines the available evidence supporting the complex relationship between serum uric acid (sUA) and heart failure (HF).

Recently published literature indicates that hyperuricemia is a risk factor, as well as a risk marker for cardiovascular diseases. High sUA levels correlate with an increased risk of incident HF in community adults, and this incidence is related to hyperuricemia severity.

Hyperuricemia is common in established HF with reduced ejection fraction, with a higher prevalence in severely symptomatic patients. Elevated sUA levels are a prognostic marker, predicting adverse outcomes in terms of mortality and rehospitalization for acute HF and severe chronic systolic and diastolic HF. The responsible mechanisms for the deleterious effects of high uric acid levels in cardiovascular disease and the uric acid paradox will be briefly reviewed. The increased production of free oxygen radicals as a consequence of elevated xanthine-

* Corresponding author: Adriana Ilieşiu, MD, PhD, FESC. Department of Internal Medicine and Cardiology, "Carol Davila" University of Medicine and Pharmacy, "Theodor Burghele" Clinical Hospital, Bucharest, Romania. E-mail: adilies@yahoo.com.

oxidase activity provides the basis for urate lowering therapy. Recent evidence and conflicting results related to urate lowering therapy with xanthine-oxidase inhibitors will also be summarized.

INTRODUCTION

Heart failure (HF) bears high morbi-mortality and a substantial economic burden, despite major advances in the disease treatment during the last decades [1, 2]. Complex pathophysiologic mechanisms, e.g., neurohormonal activation, inflammation and increased oxidative stress, are involved in left ventricular remodeling, contributing to HF progression.

The association of serum uric acid (sUA) with incident and established HF, as well as with cardiovascular conditions leading to HF (arterial hypertension, atherosclerosis) has been demonstrated by many epidemiological, clinical and experimental data. This relationship was noticed not only in hyperuricemia, but also in high - normal sUA levels (sUA > 5.5 mg/dl) [3, 4]. There is available evidence suggesting that sUA is both a risk factor and a marker of HF severity, hyperuricemia is associated with enhanced oxidative stress, and the direct deleterious effects of sUA contribute to HF progression.

sUA AND INCIDENT HF

The association between hyperuricemia, as a risk factor, and incident HF has been prospectively addressed in various studies.

In the Framingham Offspring cohort, the relationship between baseline sUA level and subsequent HF development has been analyzed in a group of young (mean baseline age 36 years, women 52%) general community dwellers. After 29 years median follow-up and the cumulative observation time of 135,991 person-years, the incidence rates of HF were approximately 6-fold higher among those at the highest quartile of sUA (>6.3 mg/dL) compared to those at the lowest quartile (<3.4 mg/dL) [5]. In this large prospective study, hyperuricemia emerged as a novel, independent risk factor for the development of HF.

The association between hyperuricemia and incident HF among older adults was evaluated in the Cardiovascular Health Study. In 5461 adults ≥65 years after 8,1 years of mean follow-up, incident HF occurred in 21%

participants with hyperuricemia compared to 18% participants without hyperuricemia. Each 1 mg/dl increase in sUA was associated with 12% increase in incident HF. sUA was associated with an increased risk of incident, new-onset HF, with a hazard ratio (HR) 1.30 (95% confidence interval (CI) 1.05-1.60) among hyperuricemic subjects versus normals per 1 mg/dl increase [6]. Interestingly, the data from the subgroups analysis indicates that in patients with renal disease, hypertension, hyperinsulinemia or thiazides diuretic treatment, despite having a higher sUA level, there was no association between hyperuricemia and incident HF [7]. These data suggest that sUA may predict new-onset HF only when it is a marker of increased XO activity, hypothesizing a lack of direct sUA effects.

In a recent meta-analysis of different studies on community-based populations, health check-ups, outpatients and patients with coronary artery disease, 427 917 participants between 36 and 73 years old were included [8]. The odds of HF development increased by 19% (HR 1.19, 95% CI 1.17-1.21) for every 1 mg/dL increase in sUA. Furthermore, a dose–effect relationship between sUA and incident HF has been demonstrated.

In summary, high sUA was found to be associated with increased incidence of HF, particularly when hyperuricemia was a marker of increased oxidative stress, in many large prospective studies.

PREVALENCE OF HYPERURICEMIA IN ESTABLISHED HF

Elevated serum uric acid is common in preexisting HF and its prevalence varies according to the characteristics of HF patients and the threshold for defining hyperuricemia [9, 10, 11].

In a retrospective cohort study, 37% of 6204 patients with HF had sUA > 7 mg/dl. sUA levels were higher in younger men, in patients with ischemic heart disease, diabetes mellitus and hypertension [12]. At baseline, sUA was mostly influenced by impaired renal function urea and diuretic treatment and increased in almost half of the patients after 27 months follow-up. In the Japanese Cardiac Registry of Heart Failure in Cardiology, 56% of 1869 patients had hyperuricemia defined by serum uric acid ≥7 mg/dl [13]. The Beta-Blocker Evaluation of Survival Trial (BEST) included 2645 patients with severe left and right ventricular systolic dysfunction. Hyperuricemia was defined by sUA level ≥8 mg/dL for men and ≥6 mg/dL for women. In this high-risk chronic HF population/cohort, 54% of patients had hyperuricemia and the mean sUA level was 9.2 mg/dL [14].

Acute HF is a distinct entity with high prevalence of signs of systemic and pulmonary congestion, cardiorenal syndrome and diuretic use. In the Efficacy of Vasopressin Antagonism in Heart Failure Outcome Study With Tolvaptan (EVEREST) trial, in a large cohort of 3955 patients hospitalized for acute decompensated HF with low EF, aproximately 50% had elevated sUA. The mean sUA value was 9,1 mg/dl and higher sUA levels were associated with more severe functional class, systolic dysfunction, lower systolic pressure and impairement of renal function [15].

Increased sUA levels are also associated with HF with preserved ejection fraction (EF), a HF entity which constitutes approximately half of all HF patients. In 300 patients hospitalized for decompensated HF, several biomarkers were compared between patients with reduced and preserved EF. Patients with HF with preserved EF had similar increase in sUA levels as patients with HF with low EF, with a mean sUA value of 9.5 mg/dl. Hyperuricemia remained unchanged in both groups after 60 days [16]. In another study, 59% out of 424 patients hospitalized for decompensated HF with preserved EF had hyperuricemia (sUA > 7 mg/dl) [17]. Compared to normouricemic patients, hyperuricemic patients had a higher prevalence of hypertension, diabetes mellitus, dyslipidemia, atrial fibrillation and diuretic use.

There is a growing evidence that higher sUA values are associated with worsening of HF functional class and hemodynamic parameters of HF severity. Hyperuricemic patients were more symptomatic and the mean duration of HF was longer [14, 18]. sUA was inversely associated with functional capacity and maximal oxygen consumption in HF patients with low, as well in patients with preserved EF [17, 19]. Patients with end-stage CHF and cachectic patients had higher sUA levels, partly as a consequence of increased catabolism with increased substrate for UA synthesis [11, 20].

sUA level was associated with lower left ventricular systolic function estimated by EF, both in stable and worsening HF [12, 15].

The relationship between sUA and left ventricular EF and NT-proBNP levels has been demonstrated [15, 21, 22, 23, 24]. Hyperuricaemia has also been found to be a marker of pulmonary and systemic congestion, being related to the severity of diastolic dysfunction and elevated filling pressures, both in patients with HF with reduced and preserved EF [12, 17, 24, 25, 26, 27, 28, 29].

Therefore, elevated sUA is frequently associated with severe chronic and acute decompensated cardiac failure and appears as a marker of HF severity.

PATHOPHYSIOLOGY OF INCREASED SUA IN HF

Many factors contribute to hyperuricemia, however increased UA production, decreased renal excretion, or a combination of both are the main mechanisms in the setting of HF.

UA is the final oxidation product of purine catabolism in humans. The conversion of hypoxanthine to UA is the last metabolic step and is regulated by xanthine oxidoreductase (XOR). As XO uses molecular oxygen as an electron acceptor, this process generates superoxide anion and hydrogen peroxide and contributes to reactive oxygen and nitrogen species formation. Also, the liver and the small intestine are the major sources of XOR, in cardiovascular diseases there is evidence for activation of XO pathway and increased UA production in the capillary vascular and myocardial endothelial cells [31, 31]. Tissue hypoxia and increased catabolic state in HF lead to the accumulation of UA precursors, hypoxanthine and xanthine, increasing XO substrate. XOR up-regulation and the increased conversion to XO also contributes to UA synthesis. In HF patients, the endothelium-bound XOR activity was enhanced >200% compared with controls [32, 33].

The impairment of UA renal excretion occurs in patients with chronic kidney disease, hypertension, hyperinsulinemia and thiazide diuretic treatment, increasing sUA level despite normal UA synthesis. Decreased glomerular filtration rate and increased UA tubular absorption generated by increased norepinephrine and angiotensin II levels are the main mechanisms. Chronic diuretic use lowers urate excretion and increases tubular UA reabsorption, further increasing sUA [18, 34, 35]. The co-existence of renal failure is a common cause of hyperuricemia, patients with HF and severe renal dysfunction having the highest sUA levels [13, 18].

However, in many clinical HF studies the prognostic value of hyperuricemia remains significant after adjustment for confounding factors, especially renal function and insulin resistance, suggesting that up-regulation of XO activity and increased UA synthesis are the dominating factors. Thus, hyperuricemia is mainly a marker of XO activation generating oxidants during UA production with many deleterious effects on vascular and cardiac function [9, 36].

UA may activate the inflammatory pathway and stimulation of cytokines (e.g., monocyte chemoattractant protein-1). A correlation between sUA and C-reactive protein, inflammatory cytokines, IL-6, TNF alpha, adhesion molecules and their soluble receptors has been demonstrated in HF patients. sUA emerged as a strong predictor for inflammatory response, independent of diuretic dose, and serum creatinine and its levels parallel the chronic inflammatory response which occurs with increasing CHF severity [24, 37, 38, 39, 40]. Increased reactive oxygen species (ROS) formation and inflammatory immune activation may further contribute to increased XO activity completing the vicious circle between inflammation, oxidative stress and UA overproduction [41].

The mechanism linking UA, inflammatory markers and vasoconstrictive pathways activation occurs inside the cells, where UA is uptaken via organic anion transporters. At the intracellular level UA is pro-oxidant, inducing oxidative stress in the mitochondria, mitochondrial dysfunction and activation of NADPH [42, 43, 44]. Intracellular UA activates the specific mitogen activated protein kinases and nuclear transcription factors, leading to activation of vasoconstrictive mediators, angiotensin II, thromboxane and endothelin-1 [42, 45, 46, 47, 48, 49].

HF patients have significant endothelial dysfunction with vasodilatation impairment and decreased exercise tolerance [50]. Endothelial dysfunction is partially mediated by oxidative stress, which disrupts the normal NO signaling and reduces NO bioavailability either by the direct effect of UA itself, or by activation of angiotensin II [42, 48, 52, 53, 54, 55, 56].

The XOR up-regulation in the failing myocardium has multiple deleterious effects and contributes to the myocardial dysfunction, ROS-induced myocardial damage and to the myocardial fibrosis [57, 58]. Increased oxidative stress impairs myocardial contractility enhancing oxygen consumption at the level of myofilament and myocardium, decreases the mechano-energetic coupling and alters calcium sensitivity [59, 60, 61, 62, 63]. XO impairs mechano-energetic coupling by interacting with NO signaling systems, partly in the sarcoplasmic reticulum of myocytes [64]. The increased transcardiac gradient of UA between the coronary sinus and aorta has been demonstrated in patients with chronic HF, suggesting that high plasma UA level is partly secreted from the failing heart [65].

The sUA paradox consists in the dual role of UA, which can act either as an anti-oxidant or a pro-oxidant. There is an ongoing debate about the role of UA as contributing to or preventing the adverse effects in HF patients.

sUA is a powerful antioxidant, protecting against free radical damage. Along with ascorbate, sUA accounts for up to 60% of serum free radical scavenging capacity. Under conditions of oxidative stress, the reduced endothelial NO activity increases XO activity and acutely elevates sUA [66, 67]. sUA reacts with superoxide, peroxinitrite and with NO, protecting vascular endothelial cells from external oxidative stress [55, 68, 69, 70, 71].

The acute infusion of exogenous UA into the extracellular circulatory system improved endothelial function [72, 73]. However, in these studies the protective UA effect was obtained at high doses of exogenous UA. In HF, the endogenous UA overproduction with hyperuricemia has detrimental effects due to hypoxia-induced XO upregulation, increased ROS accumulation and to the direct deleterious effect of UA inside the cells [42, 43, 44].

The Prognostic Role of sUA in HF Patients

The prognostic role of hyperuricemia in patients with HF was reported in many clinical studies. Furthermore, sUA is included in the Seattle HF Model prognostic score [74].

In a prospective study, in patients with moderate to severe chronic HF and low EF, high sUA was a strong and independent metabolic marker predicting mortality and need for heart transplantation [9]. There was a gradual relationship between sUA and mortality, the cutoff value of 9.5 mg/dL being found as the best predictor of mortality at 12 months. When associated with hemodynamic (EF) and functional status (maximal oxygen consumption with exercise), the severity of hyperuricemia added prognostic information. For a higher number of risk factors the mortality increases, reaching a 3 year mortality of 87.5% in patients with all three risk factors.

In another study, high plasma sUA emerged as an independent prognostic factor for mortality, along with other conventional factors such as natriuretic peptide and renal function in patients with chronic HF and reduced EF. sUA, partly secreted by the dysfunctional myocardium, increased with the severity of chronic HF [65].

In the randomized trial to determine the effect of nebivolol on mortality and cardiovascular hospital admission in elderly patients with heart failure (SENIORS) trial, the dataset of 2128 elderly HF patients (≥70 years) was used to establish a risk prediction score using a multivariate model. In addition to traditional prognostic markers, sUA emerged as a relevant prognostic marker for all-cause mortality and new HF readmission [75].

Not only baseline hyperuricemia (sUA > 7.7 mg/dL), but also sUA increase during follow-up were independent predictors of increased mortality and increased cardiac hospitalizations in patients with HF [12].

The prognostic value of hyperuricaemia in patients hospitalized for acute decompensated HF has been reported [18]. During 24 months follow-up after having been hospitalized for acute HF with reduced EF, patients with hyperuricemia had higher risk of death and new HF readmission. sUA emerged as an independent long-term prognostic marker in addition to age, HF functional class and cardiac function.

The evaluation of sUA as a risk marker for all-cause mortality and the assessment of sUA cut-off for the increase in risk were analysed in a meta-analysis including data from six studies of 1456 patients with HF with low EF [76]. sUA was found to be a prognostic marker, with a liniar association between sUA level >7 mg/dL and all-cause mortality.

In a recent prospective observational study focusing on HF patients with preserved EF, the relationship between sUA and mortality was analyzed [17]. 424 consecutive patients hospitalized for decompensated HFpEF were divided into two groups based on the presence of hyperuricemia (serum uric acid ≥7 mg/dl or taking antihyperuricemic agents). Hyperuricemia was an independent predictor of all-cause mortality after adjustment for several confounding factors including chronic kidney disease and use of diuretics. The authors' conclusion was that in patients with HF with preserved EF the presence of hyperuricemia indicates advanced arterial stiffness and impaired exercise capacity associated with increased mortality.

However, some studies emphasize the different prognostic role of hyperuricemia in patients with HF based on the mechanism of sUA increase, overproduction vs decreased renal excretion due to renal dysfunction.

In the Beta-Blocker Evaluation of Survival Trial (BEST), hyperuricemia and its outcomes were evaluated in patients with moderate-severe chronic HF [14]. The association between hyperuricemia and all-cause mortality and HF hospitalization was noted only in patients with normal renal function (eGFR > 60 mL/min/1.73 m^2). In patients with chronic kidney disease, although the prevalence of hyperuricemia and the mean sUA level were significantly higher, the association was no longer significant.

The relationship between sUA and outcomes was compared across sUA quartile in the EVEREST trial, in a large cohort of 3955 patients hospitalized for worsening chronic HF with low EF [15]. Baseline sUA was a strong and independent prognostic marker of a worse outcome (all-cause mortality and a composite of cardiovascular mortality or HF hospitalization) only in patients with preserved baseline renal function (eGFR ≥ 30 ml/min/1.73 m^2).

The prognostic impact and the determinants of hyperuricemia in hospitalized patients with acute HF were analyzed in a Japanese study using the data drawn from an intramural registry [77]. There was a 43% mortality in the 1,835 elderly patients (mean age 75 ± 13 years) during 27 months median follow-up. The major determinants of sUA levels were renal function and perfusion and left ventricular EF. sUA was a significant predictor of mortality for acute HF with either reduced or preserved EF, with an increasing risk of death along the quartile distribution of sUA. However, the prognostic significance of hyperuricemia on long-term mortality diminished with worsening renal function.

These epidemiological studies suggest that the prognostic significance of sUA in patients with acute and chronic HF is linked to the pathophysiologic mechanism of sUA increase. Hyperuricemia due to overproduction, marker of XO up-regulation and increased oxidative stress, rather than hyperuricemia resulting from decreased renal clearance alone is associated with poor outcomes in HF patients.

TREATMENT WITH XO INHIBITORS IN HF

sUA overproduction as a marker of XO activity up-regulation provides the rationale for using XO inhibitors on top of conventional HF treatment, in order to improve the outcome of HF patients.

Experimental studies with allopurinol and oxypurinol have shown beneficial effects on cardiac and vascular function. XO inhibition treatment decreased myocardial oxygen consumption, improving mechano-energetic coupling, preventing LV remodeling, and improving LV systolic function [61, 63, 78, 79].

In 16 patients with idiopathic dilated cardiomyopathy, intracoronary infusion of allopurinol decreased myocardial oxygen consumption, while maintaining dP/dt and stroke work [60]. The concentration and the rate of adenosine triphosphate synthesis through creatine kinase, measured by magnetic resonance spectroscopy, were acutely increased by intravenous infusion of allopurinol in patients with non-ischemic cardiomyopathy [80]. These results suggest the improvement of the energetic imbalance in the failing myocardium under XO inhibition treatment. Short-term allopurinol treatment had beneficial effects on left ventricular systolic and diastolic function and on coronary flow reserve in patients with HF [81, 82].

The vascular benefits of XO inhibition on peripheral blood flow and endothelial function have been evaluated. In hyperuricemic patients with HF, acute and chronic allopurinol treatment improved endothelium-dependent vasodilation and increased peak blood flow. There was a direct relationship between blood flow increase and changes in sUA [70]. The effect of allopurinol on endothelial function generated a steep dose-response curve, and was related to the reduction in vascular oxidative stress, since the urate-lowering drug probenecid had no effect on endothelial function for similar urate lowering rates [83].

Small interventional clinical studies have shown beneficial effects of XO inhibitors in HF patients. Allopurinol improved EF and reduced B-type natriuretic peptide in patients with chronic HF [81, 85]. The uricosuric treatment with benzbromarone, despite significantly decreasing sUA, failed to improve left ventricular EF, B-type natriuretic peptide and NYHA functional class in patients with chronic HF and hyperuricemia [86]. These results support the hypothesis that XO up-regulation rather than hyperuricemia explains the association between sUA and HF prognosis.

Allopurinol treatment was independently associated with improved survival at 1.4 years follow-up in a retrospective HF study [12]. Other observational studies in HF patients with gout suggest that treatment with allopurinol had beneficial effects on survival [87, 88].

The efficacy of XO inhibition on top of optimal HF treatment on prognosis and quality of life was assessed in patients with chronic HF and reduced EF in two large prospective studies [23, 89]. In The Impact of Oxypurinol in Patients With Symptomatic Heart Failure (OPT-CHF) study the efficacy of oxypurinol 600 mg/day on morbidity, mortality, and quality of life was evaluated in 405 patients with moderate-severe CHF and reduced EF. The treatment with oxypurinol had no clinical benefit in unselected HF patients at 6 months. However, in a post hoc analysis, a subgroup of hyperuricemic patients with sUA level ≥9.5 mg/dl improved their clinical status, the favorable clinical outcome correlating with the degree of sUA reduction.

The hypothesis of the Xanthine Oxidase Inhibition for Hyperuricemic Heart Failure Patients (EXACT-HF) study was that treatment with high-dose allopurinol would improve clinical outcome in patients with symptomatic chronic HF, systolic dysfunction and hyperuricemia (≥9.5 mg/dl). 253 patients with HF NYHA class II-IV, low EF (median EF of 25%) and sUA level ≥9.5 mg/dl were treated with allopurinol 600 mg/day for 24 weeks. Although uric acid levels decreased by ≈45%, XO inhibition with high-dose allopurinol did not improve any of the end-points (clinical status, quality of life, exercise capacity and left ventricular function) at 6 months, in these hyperuricemic high-risk chronic HF patients. Similar to OPT-CHF results, there was a trend toward reduced HF hospitalizations at 6 months. High doses allopurinol were well tolerated and safe, even in HF patients with concomitant renal dysfunction.

The authors comment on the study results, pointing out the possible explanations for the lack of benefit of high-dose allopurinol in chronic HF patients. Treatment failure could be related to the high-risk profile of HF population, the study duration and the complexity of HF pathophysiological mechanisms. The patients were symptomatic for an average of 5 years, with significant impairment in clinical status and frequent hospitalizations for acute HF decompensation despite optimal guideline recommended therapy and had multiple co-morbidities. The cumulative rate of events was high, around 40% for death or all-cause hospitalization at 24 weeks. Considering the trend toward reduced HF hospitalizations at 24 weeks, the hypothesis that a longer treatment with high-dose allopurinol could have significant beneficial effects on HF morbi-mortality cannot be refuted. Another explanation for XO inhibition inefficiency could be related to the different pathophysiological HF mechanisms involved in HF progression, such as oxidative stress pathways independent of XO inhibition or inflammation with activation of proinflammatory cytokines leading to hyperuricemia [90].

To sum up, despite positive effects in pre-clinical experimental work, small clinical mechanicistic studies and retrospective epidemiological studies, randomized clinical trials have documented no beneficial effects of XO-inhibition on clinical status, functional capacity, quality of life and cardiac function in hyperuricemic chronic HF patients with systolic dysfunction.

CONCLUSION

The epidemiological data emphasize the high prevalence of hyperuricemia in HF and qualifies sUA as a biological marker of disease severity along with other established clinical, hemodynamic and metabolic markers.

Although multiple factors contribute to the increase of sUA levels, overproduction or impaired excretion are the main mechanisms involved in HF- associated hyperuricemia. However, a growing body of evidence suggests that increased sUA production due to hypoxia and high catabolic rate are prevalent in chronic HF in contrast to gout, where impaired renal excretion is the dominant source of hyperuricemia.

Increased sUA synthesis as a marker of XO up-regulation and increased oxidative stress are predictive for HF development and convey a negative prognosis in established HF. sUA overproduction contributes to HF progression, having a negative impact on survival, hospitalization, symptoms and exercise capacity in patients with HF. Therefore, sUA proves to be a useful risk marker, readily accessible and at a low cost, offering relevant prognostic information in HF patients.

The treatment with XO inhibitors, despite pathophysiological hypothesis generating and promising results in experimental and small clinical studies, failed to show beneficial effects in patients with HF and reduced EF in large prospective, randomized trials. Therefore, in the present guidelines, the treatment with XO inhibitors is only indicated in HF with reduced EF associated with gout [91].

Nevertheless, high dose allopurinol deserves further trials in other cardiovascular diseases in the cardiovascular continuum, such as hypertension, diabetes mellitus or ischemic heart disease associated with potential progression to HF.

References

[1] Lindenfeld J, Albert NM, Boehmer JP, Collins SP, Ezekowitz JA, Givertz MM, Katz SD, Klapholz M, Moser DK, Rogers JG, Starling RC, Stevenson WG, Tang WH, Teerlink JR, Walsh MN. HFSA 2010 Comprehensive Heart Failure Practice Guideline. *J. Card. Fail.* 2010 Jun;16(6):e1-194. doi: 10.1016/j.cardfail.2010.04.004.

[2] Levantesi G, Marfisi RM, Franzosi MG, Maggioni AP, Nicolosi GL, Schweiger C, Silletta MG, Tavazzi L, Tognoni G, Marchioli R. Uric acid: a cardiovascular risk factor in patients with recent myocardial infarction. *Int. J. Cardiol.* 2013 Jul. 15;167(1):262-9.

[3] Niskanen LK, Laaksonen DE, Nyyssönen K, Alfthan G, Lakka HM, Lakka TA, Salonen JT. Uric acid level as a risk factor for cardiovascular and all-cause mortality in middle-aged men: a prospective cohort study. *Arch. Intern. Med.* 2004 Jul. 26;164(14):1546-51.

[4] Feig DI, Kang DH, Johnson RJ. Uric acid and cardiovascular risk. *N. Engl. J. Med.* 2008 Oct. 23;359(17):1811-21. doi: 10.1056/NEJMra0800 885.

[5] Krishnan E. Hyperuricemia and incident heart failure. *Circ. Heart Fail.* 2009 Nov;2(6):556-62.

[6] Ekundayo OJ, Dell'Italia LJ, Sanders PW, Arnett D, Aban I, Love TE, Filippatos G, Anker SD, Lloyd-Jones DM, Bakris G, Mujib M, Ahmed A. Association between hyperuricemia and incident heart failure among older adults: a propensity-matched study. *Int. J. Cardiol.* 2010 Jul. 23; 142(3):279-87. doi: 10.1016/j.ijcard.2009.01.010. Epub. 2009 Feb. 6.

[7] Desai RV, Ahmed MI, Fonarow GC, Filippatos GS, White M, Aban IB, Aronow WS, Ahmed A. Effect of serum insulin on the association between hyperuricemia and incident heart failure. *Am. J. Cardiol.* 2010 Oct. 15;106(8):1134-8. doi: 10.1016/j.amjcard.2010.06.023.

[8] Huang H, Huang B, Li Y, Huang Y, Li J, Yao H, Jing X, Chen J, Wang J. Uric acid and risk of heart failure: a systematic review and meta-analysis. *Eur. J. Heart Fail.* 2014 Jan;16(1):15-24. doi: 10.1093/eurjhf/hft132. Epub. 2013 Dec. 3.

[9] Anker SD, Doehner W, Rauchhaus M, Sharma R, Francis D, Knosalla C, Davos CH, Cicoira M, Shamim W, Kemp M, Segal R, Osterziel KJ, Leyva F, Hetzer R, Ponikowski P, Coats AJ. Uric acid and survival in chronic HF: validation and application in metabolic, functional, and hemodynamic staging. *Circulation.* 2003 Apr. 22;107(15):1991-7.

[10] Kittleson MM, St John ME, Bead V, Champion HC, Kasper EK, Russell SD, Wittstein IS, Hare JM. Increased levels of uric acid predict haemodynamic compromise in patients with heart failure independently of B-type natriuretic peptide levels. *Heart.* 2007;93:365-367.

[11] Doehner W, Rauchhaus M, Florea VG, Sharma R, Bolger AP, Davos CH, Coats AJS, Anker SD. Uric acid in cachectic and noncachectic patients with chronic HF: relationship to leg vascular resistance. *Am. Heart J.* 2001; 141:792-9.

[12] Gotsman I, Keren A, Lotan C, Zwas DR. Changes in uric acid levels and allopurinol use in chronic heart failure: association with improved survival. *J. Card. Fail.* 2012:18;694-701.

[13] Hamaguchi S, Furumoto T, Tsuchihashi-Makaya M, Goto K, Goto D, Yokota T, Kinugawa S, Yokoshiki H, Takeshita A, Tsutsui H; JCARE-CARD Investigators. Hyperuricemia predicts adverse outcomes in patients with heart failure. *Int. J. Cardiol.* 2011 Sep. 1;151(2):143-7. doi: 10.1016/j.ijcard.2010.05.002. Epub. 2010 Jun. 14.

[14] Filippatos GS, Ahmed MI, Gladden JD, Mujib M, Aban IB, Love TE, Sanders PW, Pitt B, Anker SD, Ahmed A. Hyperuricaemia, chronic kidney disease, and outcomes in heart failure: potential mechanistic insights from epidemiological data. *Eur. Heart J.* 2011 Mar;32(6):712-20. doi: 10.1093/eurheartj/ehq473. Epub. 2011 Jan. 3.

[15] Vaduganathan M, Greene SJ, Ambrosy AP, Mentz RJ, Subacius HP, Chioncel O, Maggioni AP, Swedberg K, Zannad F, Konstam MA, Senni M, Givertz MM, Butler J, Gheorghiade M; EVEREST trial investigators. Relation of serum uric acid levels and outcomes among patients hospitalized for worsening heart failure with reduced EF (from the

efficacy of vasopressin antagonism in heart failure outcome study with tolvaptan trial). *Am. J. Cardiol.* 2014 Dec. 1;114(11):1713-21. doi: 10. 1016/j.amjcard.2014.09.008. Epub. 2014 Sep. 16.

[16] Bishu K, Deswal A, Chen HH, LeWinter MM, Lewis GD, Semigran MJ, Borlaug BA, McNulty S, Hernandez AF, Braunwald E, Redfield MM. Biomarkers in acutely decompensated heart failure with preserved or reduced ejection fraction. *Am. Heart J.* 2012 Nov;164(5):763-770.e3. doi: 10.1016/j.ahj.2012.08.014. Epub. 2012 Oct. 16.

[17] Shimizu T, Yoshihisa A, Kanno Y, Takiguchi M, Sato A, Miura S, Nakamura Y, Yamauchi H, Owada T, Abe S, Sato T, Suzuki S, Oikawa M, Yamaki T, Sugimoto K, Kunii H, Nakazato K, Suzuki H, Saitoh S, Takeishi Y.Relationship of hyperuricemia with mortality in heart failure patients with preserved EF. *Am. J. Physiol. Heart Circ. Physiol.* 2015 Oct;309(7):H1123-9. doi: 10.1152/ajpheart.00533.2015. Epub. 2015 Aug. 21.

[18] Pascual-Figal DA, Hurtado-Martinez JA, Redondo B, Antolinos MJ, Ruiperez JA, Valdes M. Hyperuricaemia and long-term outcome after hospital discharge in acute heart failure patients. *Eur. J. Heart Fail.* 2007;9:518e524.

[19] Leyva F, Anker SD, Swan JW, Godsland IF, Wingrove CS, Chua TP, Stevenson JC, Coats AJS. Serum uric acid as an index of impaired oxidative metabolism in chronic HF. *Eur. Heart J.* 1997;18:858-65.

[20] Anker SD, Leyva F, Poole-Wilson PA, Kox WJ, Stevenson JC, Coats AJ. Relation between serum uric acid and lower limb blood flow in patients with chronic heart failure. *Heart.* 1997 Jul;78(1):39-43.

[21] Pinelli M, Bindi M, Filardo FP, Moroni F, Castiglioni M. Serum uric acid levels correlate with left ventricular EF and systolic pulmonary artery pressure in patients with HF. [Article in Italian] *Recenti Prog. Med.* 2007;98(12):619-23.

[22] Borghi C, Cosentino ER, Rinaldi ER, Cicero AF. Uricaemia and ejection fraction in elderly heart failure outpatients. *Eur. J. Clin. Invest.* 2014 Jun;44(6):573-8. doi: 10.1111/eci.12273.

[23] Hare JM, Mangal B, Brown J, Fisher C Jr, Freudenberger R, Colucci WS, Mann DL, Liu P, Givertz MM, Schwarz RP; OPT-CHF Investigators.. Impact of oxypurinol in patients with symptomatic heart failure. Results of the OPT-CHF study. *J. Am. Coll. Cardiol.* 2008; 51 (24):2301-9. DOI: 10.1016/j.jacc.2008.01.068.

[24] Iliesiu A, Campeanu A, Marta D, Parvu I, Gheorghe G. Uric Acid, Oxidative Stress and Inflammation in Chronic Heart Failure with Reduced Ejection Fraction. *Rev. Rom. Med. Lab.* 2015 Dec; 23(4); 397-406.

[25] Hoeper MM, Hohlfeld JM, Fabel H. Hyperuricaemia in patients with right or left HF. *Eur. Respir. J.* 1999;13:682-5.

[26] Cicoira M, Zanolla L, Rossi A, Golia G, Franceschini L, Brighetti G, Zeni P, Zardini P. Elevated serum uric acid levels are associated with diastolic dysfunction in patients with dilated cardiomyopathy. *Am. Heart J.* 2002; 143(6):1107-11. DOI: 10.1067/mhj.2002.122122.

[27] Zhang YH, Lü R, Zhao XY, Kang LM, Yang YJ, Zhang J. Association of serum uric acid, plasma NT-proBNP, Hs-C reactive protein and invasive hemodynamic parameters in patients with heart failure. *Zhonghua Xin Xue Guan Bing Za Zhi.* 2009;37(2):126-9.

[28] Wojciechowska C, Romuk E, Tomasik A, Skrzep-Poloczek B, Nowalany-Kozielska E, Birkner E, Jache W. Oxidative stress markers and c-reactive protein are related to severity of HF in patients with dilated cardiomyopathy. *Mediators Inflamm.* 2014;2014:147040. doi: 10. 1155/2014/147040. Epub. 2014 Oct. 23.

[29] Nogi S, Fujita S, Okamoto Y, Kizawa S, Morita H, Ito T, Sakane K, Sohmiya K, Hoshiga M, Ishizaka N. Serum uric acid is associated with cardiac diastolic dysfunction among women with preserved ejection fraction. *Am. J. Physiol. Heart Circ. Physiol.* 2015 Sep;309(5):H986-94. doi: 10.1152/ajpheart.00402.2015. Epub. 2015 Jul. 24.

[30] Jarasch ED, Grund C, Bruder G, Heid HW, Keenan TW, Franke WW. Localization of xanthine oxidase in mammary-gland epithelium and capillary endothelium. *Cell.* 1981 Jul;25(1):67-82.

[31] Nees S, Gerbes AL, Gerlach E, Staubesand J. Isolation, identification, and continuous culture of coronary endothelial cells from guinea pig hearts. *Eur. J. Cell Biol.* 1981 Jun;24(2):287-97.

[32] Hassoun PM, Shedd AL, Lanzillo JJ, Thappa V, Landman MJ, Fanburg BL. Inhibition of pulmonary artery smooth muscle cell growth by hypoxanthine, xanthine, and uric acid. *Am. J. Respir. Cell. Mol. Biol.* 1992 Jun;6(6):617-24.

[33] Landmesser U, Spiekermann S, Dikalov S, Tatge H, Wilke R, Kohler C, Harrison DG, Hornig B, Drexler H. Vascular oxidative stress and endothelial dysfunction in patients with chronic heart failure: role of xanthine-oxidase and extracellular superoxide dismutase. *Circulation.* 2002 Dec. 10;106(24):3073-8.

[34] Reyes AJ. The increase in serum UA concentration caused by diuretics might be beneficial in HF. *Eur. J. Heart Fail.* 2005 Jun;7(4):461-7.

[35] Steele TH, Oppenheimer S. Factors affecting urate excretion following diuretic administration in man. *Am. J. Med.* 1969 Oct;47(4):564-74.

[36] Berry CE, Hare JM. Xanthine oxidoreductase and cardiovascular disease: molecular mechanisms and pathophysiological implications. *J. Physiol.* 2004 Mar. 16;555(Pt 3):589-606. Epub. 2003 Dec. 23.

[37] Leyva F, Anker SD, Godsland IF, Teixeira M, Hellewell PG, Kox WJ, Poole-Wilson PA, Coats AJ. UA in chronic heart failure: a marker of chronic inflammation. *Eur. Heart J.* 1998 Dec;19(12):1814-22. DOI: 10. 1053/euhj.1998.1188.

[38] Ruggiero C, Cherubini A, Ble A, Bos AJ, Maggio M, Dixit VD, Lauretani F, Bandinelli S, Senin U, Ferrucci L. UA and inflammatory markers. *Eur. Heart J.* 2006;27:1174-81.

[39] Fröhlich M, Imhof A, Berg G, Hutchinson WL, Pepys MB, Boeing H, Muche R, Brenner H, Koenig W. Association between C-reactive protein and features of the metabolic syndrome: a population-based study. *Diabetes Care.* 2000 Dec;23(12):1835-9.

[40] Ruggiero C, Cherubini A, Miller E 3rd, Maggio M, Najjar SS, Lauretani F, Bandinelli S, Senin U, Ferrucci L. Usefulness of uric acid to predict changes in C-reactive protein and interleukin-6 in 3-year period in Italians aged 21 to 98 years. *Am. J. Cardiol.* 2007 Jul. 1;100(1):115-21. Epub. 2007 May 24.

[41] Komaki Y, Sugiura H, Koarai A, Tomaki M, Ogawa H, Akita T, Hattori T, Ichinose M. Cytokine-mediated xanthine oxidase upregulation in chronic obstructive pulmonary disease's airways. *Pulm. Pharmacol. Ther.* 2005;18(4):297-302.

[42] Yu MA, Sánchez-Lozada LG, Johnson RJ, Kang DH. Oxidative stress with an activation of the renin-angiotensin system in human vascular endothelial cells as a novel mechanism of uric acid-induced endothelial dysfunction. *J. Hypertens.* 2010 Jun;28(6):1234-42.

[43] Corry DB, Eslami P, Yamamoto K, Nyby MD, Makino H, Tuck ML. Uric acid stimulates vascular smooth muscle cell proliferation and oxidative stress via the vascular renin-angiotensin system. *J. Hypertens.* 2008 Feb;26(2):269-75. doi: 10.1097/HJH.0b013e3282f240bf.

[44] Sautin YY, Nakagawa T, Zharikov S, Johnson RJ. Adverse effects of the classic antioxidant uric acid in adipocytes: NADPH oxidase-mediated oxidative/nitrosative stress. *Am. J. Physiol. Cell. Physiol.* 2007 Aug;293 (2):C584-96. Epub. 2007 Apr. 11.

[45] Kang DH, Park SK, Lee IK, Johnson RJ. Uric acid-induced C-reactive protein expression: implication on cell proliferation and nitric oxide production of human vascular cells. *J. Am. Soc. Nephrol.* 2005;16:3553-62.

[46] Kanellis J, Watanabe S, Li JH, Kang DH, Li P, Nakagawa T, Wamsley A, Sheikh-Hamad D, Lan HY, Feng L, Johnson RJ. Uric acid stimulates monocyte chemoattractant protein-1 production in vascular smooth muscle cells via mitogen-activated protein kinase and cyclooxygenase-2. *Hypertension* 2003;41:1287-93.

[47] Watanabe S1, Kang DH, Feng L, Nakagawa T, Kanellis J, Lan H, Mazzali M, Johnson RJ. Uric acid, hominoid evolution, and the pathogenesis of salt-sensitivity. *Hypertension* 2002;40:355-60.

[48] Chao HH, Liu JC, Lin JW, Chen CH, Wu CH, Cheng TH.. Uric acid stimulates endothelin-1 gene expression associated with NADPH oxidase in human aortic smooth muscle cells. *Acta Pharmacol. Sin.* 2008;29:1301-12.

[49] Kang DH, Nakagawa T, Feng L, Watanabe S, Han L, Mazzali M, Truong L, Harris R, Johnson RJ. A role for uric acid in the progression of renal disease. *J. Am. Soc. Nephrol.* 2002;13:2888-97.

[50] Tsutsui H, Kinugawa S, Matsushima S. Oxidative stress and heart failure. *Am. J. Physiol. Heart Circ. Physiol.* 2011 Dec;301(6):H2181-90. doi: 10.1152/ajpheart.00554.2011. Epub. 2011 Sep. 23.

[51] Cirillo P, Gersch MS, Mu W, Scherer PM, Kim KM, Gesualdo L, Henderson GN, Johnson RJ, Sautin YY. Ketohexokinase-dependent metabolism of fructose induces proinflammatory mediators in proximal tubular cells. *J. Am. Soc. Nephrol.* 2009;20:545-53.

[52] Sánchez-Lozada LG, Lanaspa MA, Cristóbal-García M, García-Arroyo F, Soto V, Cruz-Robles D, Nakagawa T, Yu MA, Kang DH, Johnson RJ.. Uric acid-induced endothelial dysfunction is associated with mitochondrial alterations and decreased intracellular ATP concentrations. *Nephron Exp. Nephrol.* 2012;121:3-4.

[53] Schwartz IF, Grupper A, Chernichovski T, Grupper A, Hillel O, Engel A, Schwartz D. Hyperuricemia attenuates aortic nitric oxide generation, through inhibition of arginine transport, in rats. *J. Vasc. Res.* 2011;48: 252-60.

[54] Zharikov S, Krotova K, Hu H, Baylis C, Johnson RJ, Block ER, Patel J. Uric acid decreases NO production and increases arginase activity in cultured pulmonary artery endothelial cells. *Am. J. Physiol. Cell. Physiol.* 2008;295:C1183-90.

[55] Gersch C, Palii SP, Kim KM, Angerhofer A, Johnson RJ, Henderson GN. Inactivation of nitric oxide by uric acid. *Nucleosides Nucleotides Nucleic Acids* 2008;27:967-78.

[56] Hare JM, Stamler JS. NO/redox disequilibrium in the failing heart and cardiovascular system. *J. Clin. Invest*. 2005;115:509-17.

[57] Meerson FZ, Kagan VE, Kozlov Yu P, Belkina LM, Arkhipenko Yu V. The role of lipid peroxidation in pathogenesis of ischemic damage and the antioxidant protection of the heart. *Basic Res. Cardiol*. 1982;77:465e 85.

[58] Bendall JK, Cave AC, Heymes C, Gall N, Shah AM. Pivotal role of a gp91 (phox)-containing NADPH oxidase in angiotensin IIe induced cardiac hypertrophy in mice. *Circulation* 2002;105:293e6.

[59] Perez NG, Gao WD, Marban E. Novel myofilament Ca2fl-sensitizing property of xanthine oxidase inhibitors. *Circ. Res*. 1998 Aug. 24;83(4): 423-30.

[60] Cappola TP, Kass DA, Nelson GS, Berger RD, Rosas GO, Kobeissi ZA, Marban E, Hare JM. Allopurinol improves myocardial efficiency in patients with idiopathic dilated cardiomyopathy. *Circulation* 2001;104: 2407-11.

[61] Ekelund UE, Harrison RW, Shokek O, Thakkar RN, Tunin RS, Senzaki H, Kass DA, Marban E, Hare JM. Intravenous allopurinol decreases myocardial oxygen consumption and increases mechanical efficiency in dogs with pacing-induced heart failure. *Circ. Res*. 1999 Sep 3;85(5):437-45.

[62] Prasad K, Kalra J, Chan WP, Chaudhary AK. Effect of oxygen free radicals on cardiovascular function at organ and cellular levels. *Am. Heart J.* 1989 Jun;117(6):1196-202.

[63] Murphy RM, Dutka TL, Lamb GD. Hydroxyl radical and glutathione interactions alter calcium sensitivity and maximum force of the contractile apparatus in rat skeletal muscle fibres. *J. Physiol*. 2008 Apr. 15;586(8):2203-16. doi: 10.1113/jphysiol.2007.150516. Epub. 2008 Feb. 28.

[64] Khan SA, Lee K, Minhas KM, Gonzalez DR, Raju SVY, Tejani AD, Li D, Berkowitz DE, Hare JM. Neuronal nitric oxide synthase negatively regulates xanthine oxidoreductase inhibition of cardiac excitation-contraction coupling. *Proc. Natl. Acad. Sci. US*. 2004 Nov. 9;101(45): 15944-8. Epub. 2004 Oct. 14.

[65] Sakai H, Tsutamoto T, tsui T, Tanaka T, Ishikawa C, Horie M. Serum level of uric acid, partly secreted from the failing heart, is a prognostic

marker in patients with congestive heart failure. *Circ. J.* 2006;70:1006e 1011.

[66] Maxwell AJ, Bruinsma KA. Uric acid is closely linked to vascular nitric oxide activity. Evidence for mechanism of association with cardiovascular disease. *J. Am. Coll. Cardiol.* 2001;38:1850-8.

[67] Sevanian A, Davies KJ, Hochstein P. Serum urate as an antioxidant for ascorbic acid. *Am. J. Clin. Nutr.* 1991;54:1129S-34S.

[68] Maxwell SR, Thomason H, Sandler D, Leguen C, Baxter MA, Thorpe GH, Jones AF, Barnett AH. Antioxidant status in patients with uncomplicated insulin-dependent and non-insulin-dependent diabetes mellitus. *Eur. J. Clin. Invest.* 1997 Jun;27(6):484-90.

[69] Kuzkaya N, Weissmann N, Harrison DG, Dikalov S. Interactions of peroxynitrite with UA in the presence of ascorbate and thiols: implications for uncoupling endothelial nitric oxide synthase. *Biochem. Pharmacol.* 2005 Aug. 1;70(3):343-54.

[70] Doehner W, Schoene N, Rauchhaus M, Leyva-Leon F, Pavitt DV, Reaveley DA, Schuler G, Coats AJ, Anker SD, Hambrecht R. Effects of xanthine oxidase inhibition with allopurinol on endothelial function and peripheral blood flow in hyperuricemic patients with chronic HF: results from 2 placebo controlled studies. *Circulation* 2002;105:2619-24.

[71] Gersch C, Palii SP, Imaram W, Kim KM, Karumanchi SA, Angerhofer A, Johnson RJ, Henderson GN. Reactions of peroxynitrite with uric acid: formation of reactive intermediates, alkylated products and triuret, and in vivo production of triuret under conditions of oxidative stress. *Nucleosides Nucleotides Nucleic Acids* 2009;28:118-49.

[72] Waring WS, Convery A, Mishra V, Shenkin A, Webb DJ, Maxwell SR. Uric acid reduces exercise-induced oxidative stress in healthy adults. *Clin. Sci.* (Lond.) 2003;105:425-30.

[73] Waring WS, McKnight JA, Webb DJ, Maxwell SR. Uric acid restores endothelial function in patients with type 1 diabetes and regular smokers. *Diabetes* 2006; 55:3127-32.

[74] Levy WC, Mozaffarian D, Linker DT, Sutradhar SC, Anker SD, Cropp AB, Anand I, Maggioni A, Burton P, Sullivan MD, Pitt B, Poole-Wilson PA, Mann DL, Packer M. The Seattle Heart Failure Model: prediction of survival in heart failure. *Circulation.* 2006 Mar. 21;113(11):1424-33. Epub. 2006 Mar. 13.

[75] Manzano L, Babalis D, Roughton M, Shibata M, Anker SD, Ghio S, van Veldhuisen DJ, Cohen-Solal A, Coats AJ, Poole-Wilson PP, Flather MD; SENIORS Investigators. Predictors of clinical outcomes in elderly

patients with heart failure. *Eur. J. Heart Fail.* 2011 May;13(5):528-36. doi: 10.1093/eurjhf/hfr030. Epub. 2011 Mar. 30.

[76] Tamariz L, Harzand A, Palacio A, Verma S, Jones J, Hare J. Uric acid as a predictor of all-cause mortality in heart failure: a meta-analysis. *Congest. Heart Fail.* 2011 Jan-Feb;17(1):25-30. doi: 10.1111/j.1751-7133.2011.00200.x. Epub. 2011 Jan. 27.

[77] Huang WM, Hsu PF, Cheng HM, Lu DY, Cheng YL, Guo CY, Sung SH, Yu WC, Chen CH. Determinants and Prognostic Impact of Hyperuricemia in Hospitalization for Acute Heart Failure. *Circ. J.* 2016; 80(2):404-10. doi: 10.1253/circj.CJ-15-0964. Epub. 2015 Nov. 20.

[78] Mellin V, Isabelle M, Oudot A, Vergely-Vandriesse C, Monteil C, Di Meglio B, Henry JP, Detreaux B, Rochette L, Thuillez C, Mulder P. Transient reduction in myocardial free oxygen radical levels is involved in the improved cardiac function and structure after long-term allopurinol treatment initiated in established chronic heart failure. *Eur. Heart J.* 2005;26:1544-1550.

[79] Ukai T, Cheng CP, Tachibana H, Igawa A, Zhang ZS, Cheng HJ, Little WC. Allopurinol enhances the contractile response to dobutamine and exercise in dogs with pacing-induced heart failure. *Circulation* 2001; 103:750-755.

[80] Hirsch GA, Bottomley PA, Gerstenblith G, Weiss RG. Allopurinol acutely increases adenosine triphospate energy delivery in failing human hearts. *J. Am. Coll. Cardiol.* 2012 Feb/28;59(9):802-8. doi: 10.1016/j. jacc.2011.10.895.

[81] Cingolani HE, Plastino JA, Escudero EM, Mangal B, Brown J, P.rez NG. The effect of xanthine oxidase inhibition upon ejection fraction in heart failure patients: La Plata Study. *J. Card. Fail.* 2006;12:491-8.

[82] Erdogan D, Tayyar S, Uysal BA, Icli A, Karabacak M, Ozaydin M, Dogan A. Effects of allopurinol on coronary microvascular and left ventricular function in patients with idiopathic dilated cardiomyopathy. *Can. J. Cardiol.* 2012;28:721-7.

[83] George J, Carr E, Davies J, Belch JJ, Struthers A. High-dose allopurinol improves endothelial function by profoundly reducing vascular oxidative stress and not by lowering uric acid. *Circulation* 2006;114:2508-2516.

[84] Gavin AD, Struthers AD. Allopurinol reduces B-type natriuretic peptide concentrations and haemoglobin but does not alter exercise capacity in chronic HF. *Heart* 2005;91:749-5.

[85] Iliesiu A, Campeanu A, Marta D, Uscoiu G, Parvu I, Ciobanu A, Jinga M, Gheorghe G. Effects of high doses of allopurinol on serum uric acid

and cardiac biomarkers in chronic heart failure. *Farmacia*. 2015, Vol. 63, 4, 561-7.

[86] Ogino K, Kato M, Furuse Y, Kinugasa Y, Ishida K, Osaki S, KinugawaT, Igawa O, Hisatome I, Shigemasa C, Anker SD, Doehner W. Uric acid lowering treatment with benzbromarone in patients with heart failure: a double-blind placebo-controlled crossover preliminary study. *Circ. Heart Fail*. 2010;3:73-81.

[87] Thanassoulis G, Brophy JM, Richard H, Pilote L. Gout, allopurinol use, and heart failure outcomes. *Arch. Intern. Med*. 2010;170:1358-64.

[88] Málek F, Ošťádal P, Pařenica J, Jarkovský J, Vítovec J, Widimský P, Linhart A, Fedorco M, Coufal Z, Miklík R, Krűger A, Vondraková D, Špinar J. Uric acid, allopurinol therapy, and mortality in patients with acute heart failure--results of the Acute HEart FAilure Database registry. *J. Crit. Care*. 2012 Dec;27(6):737.e11-24. doi: 10.1016/j.jcrc.2012.03.011. Epub. 2012 Jun. 12.

[89] Givertz MM, Anstrom KJ, Redfield MM, Deswal A, Haddad H, Butler J, Tang WH, Dunlap ME, LeWinter MM, Mann DL, Felker GM, O'Connor CM, Goldsmith SR, Ofili EO, Saltzberg MT, Margulies KB, Cappola TP, Konstam MA, Semigran MJ, McNulty SE, Lee KL, Shah MR, Hernandez AF; NHLBI Heart Failure Clinical Research Network. *Circulation*. 2015 May 19;131(20):1763-71.

[90] Karantalis V, Schulman IH, Hare JM. Nitroso-redox imbalance affects cardiac structure and function. *J. Am. Coll. Cardiol*. 2013;61:933-935. doi: 10.1016/j.jacc.2012.12.016.

[91] Ponikowski P, Voors AA, Anker SD, Bueno H, Cleland JG, Coats AJ, Falk V, González-Juanatey JR, Harjola VP, Jankowska EA, Jessup M, Linde C,Nihoyannopoulos P, Parissis JT, Pieske B, Riley JP, Rosano GM, Ruilope LM, Ruschitzka F, Rutten FH, van der Meer P; Authors/Task Force Members; Document Reviewers. 2016 ESC Guidelines for the diagnosis and treatment of acute and chronic heart failure: The Task Force for the diagnosis and treatment of acute and chronic heart failure of the European Society of Cardiology (ESC). Developed with the special contribution of the Heart Failure Association (HFA) of the ESC. *Eur. J. Heart Fail*. 2016 Aug;18(8):891-975. doi: 10.1002/ejhf.592.

In: Uric Acid
Editor: Mary Newman

ISBN: 978-1-53610-287-1

Chapter 3

SERUM URIC ACID IN ACUTE HEART FAILURE SYNDROMES

Alexandru Campeanu, Adriana Iliesiu, Madalina Ababei and Tiberiu Nanea
"Carol Davila" University of Medicine and Pharmacy,
"Theodor Burghele" Clinical Hospital, Department of Internal Medicine and Cardiology, Bucharest, Romania

ABSTRACT

Acute decompensated heart failure (ADHF) is a family of related disorders, being defined as the new onset or recurrence of gradually or rapidly developing symptoms and signs of HF resulting in hospitalization and requiring urgent optimized therapy. ADHF has increasing incidence and poor prognosis, being a major cause for death and hospital readmission.

Hyperuricaemia is commonly found in patients with ADHF and has two main causes: an increase of the uric acid production because of higher abundance of purines and reduced renal function clearance, due to renal function impairment and/or diuretics treatment.

Most purines are metabolized by xanthine-oxidase (XO) particularly during hypoxia, acidosis and inflammation (present in ADHF). During this process, reactive oxygen species (ROS) are generated, leading to reduced nitric oxide release (with diminished endogenous vasodilatation and platelet aggregation) and increased oxidative stress, myocardial fibrosis, decreased cardiac muscle performance and reduced vascular tone.

Serum uric acid (sUA) may be a witness of XO upregulation, produced along with multiple ROS and may serve as a valuable biomarker for this activity in the cardiovascular system. In ADHF, the antioxidant activity of sUA demonstrated in some in-vitro studies is overcome by the pro-oxidant and pro-inflammatory effects of ROS accumulation (the sUA paradox). Hyperuricaemia was associated with greater degrees of pulmonary and systemic congestion, more vasoconstriction, and higher risk of death. Moreover, hyperuricaemia is associated with increased mortality, especially when it is a result of increased sUA production rather than decreased renal clearance.

The therapeutic approach of lowering UA levels and inhibiting XO activity can be an appealing strategy in HF. Previous studies showed that Allopurinol reduces sUA levels and myocardial oxygen consumption, improves endothelial function and reduces the serum concentration of BNP. In our recent studies with Allopurinol, we saw a significant decrease of sUA levels and significant improvements of endothelial function.

SUA, this simple, inexpensive, widely available indicator, may serve as a valuable predictive biomarker, beyond traditional prognosis markers. Adding Allopurinol to the standard treatment can be a solution for improving endothelial function in ADHF, especially for patients with hyperuricaemia.

Heart failure (HF) represents the clinical manifestation of different structural and functional cardiac and non-cardiac abnormalities. Its main consequence is the heart's inability to provide an adequate oxygen supply for ensuring a peripheral aerobic metabolism in terms of normal filling pressure, or with the cost of their increase [1].

The prevalence of HF in developed countries is 1-2% for adults, rising to more than 10% in populations over 70 years [2-5]. According to the most recent National Health and Nutrition Examination Survey, the incidence of heart failure is increasing: an estimated 5.1 million adult Americans suffer of HF and projections show that by the year 2030 the prevalence will increase by 25% [6], due to aging population and increased survival after acute pathological conditions [7].

Under the influence of some decompensation risk factor [1], such as infections, arrhythmias, decompensation of some comorbidities, lack of adherence to the treatment, patients with a history of heart failure may suffer a progressive symptomatology worsening; therefore, more than 70% of cases of acute heart failure represent the clinical worsening of chronic heart failure (acute decompensated heart failure - ADHF) [8]. Acute heart failure (AHF) is a medical emergency and is defined by rapid or gradual onset or worsening of the signs and symptoms of heart failure, requiring urgent hospitalization in order to initiate rapid treatment strategies [9].

ADHF is a heterogeneous, complex syndrome, with multiple pathophysiological mechanisms [10]. ADHF is dominated by signs of systemic congestion [11], but there is a growing body of evidence suggesting that increased oxidative stress contributes to ventricular and vascular remodeling and disease progress [12].

ADHF is a major cause of death and rehospitalization [13], having a poor prognosis [14] and being the primary cause of over a million hospitalizations annually. One of six over 65 year-olds who come to the emergency room with shortness of breath will be diagnosed with heart failure [15].

These patients are a public health burden, even after hemodynamic stabilization and discharge; secondary to progressive degradation of the cardiovascular substrate, they have an unacceptably high rate of death and rehospitalization of approximately 45% at 60 to 90 days [16] – this is the vulnerable period [17].

Cardiovascular morbidity and mortality [18] by sudden cardiac death or worsening heart failure [19] remain unacceptably high even after this period, despite therapeutic advances made in the last 30 years [20]. Thus, the overall 5-year mortality remains ≈50%, and the 1-year mortality in patients with New York Heart Association functional class III to IV HF on maximal medical therapy is 35 to 40% [21].

Given all these, there is a clear need for new parameters to predict individual prognosis and new medical solutions for a “tailored treatment” of these patients [16]. This will not only lead to clinical benefits [22], but also to smaller costs, by avoiding initiation of expensive interventions on non-responders.

Hyperuricemia is a very common metabolic disorder in the general population, with a rate of 2-18% (depending on the definition). Mean sUA levels in humans have increased gradually [23] from less than 3.5 mg/dL (210 μmol/L) in the 1920s to 6.0 to 6.5 mg/dL (360 to 390 μmol/L) in the 1970s [24]. This increase occurred simultaneously with the rapid increase of cardiovascular risk, found especially in developed countries, and is explained by changing eating habits to higher fructose and purine-rich food intake [25].

Hyperuricaemia is commonly found in patients with ADHF and has two main causes: an increase of the uric acid production because of higher abundance of purines and reduced renal function clearance, due to renal function impairment and/or diuretics treatment [26]. Oxygen pressure affects XOR gene expression. Thus, in conditions of hypoxia, acidosis or inflammation, the expression of XO increases in endothelial cells, most purines being metabolized by this isoform.

By oxidation of hypoxanthine to xanthine, and xanthine to urate, XO readily donates electrons to molecular oxygen, thereby producing superoxide radical (O2−) and hydrogen peroxide. Superoxide has been identified as the most probable ROS contributing to cardiac dysfunction in the failing myocardium [27].

The “sUA paradox” consists in the association of high sUA levels with an increased cardiovascular risk, although sUA has antioxidant properties [28]. The theory of “the anti-oxidant, pro-oxidant redox shuttle” [29] has been considered: sUA, which under normal circumstances is an anti-oxidant, becomes pro-oxidant in the atherosclerotic medium with ROS generation [30]. Also, it is conceivable that, under atherosclerotic conditions, the antioxidant activity of sUA is overcome by the pro-oxidant and pro-inflammatory effects of ROS accumulation [31].

The interaction between ROS and NO can affect cardiac function [38]. NO mediates protein S-nitrosylation at specific cysteine residues, which influences calcium flux and excitation-contraction coupling [39,40], while the interaction of O_2- with NO contributes to endothelial dysfunction by reducing NO availability [41] and produces peroxynitrite, a potent oxidant that induces apoptosis or cell necrosis [42].

Increasing imbalance between oxidative stress and decreases in the amount of nitric oxide pathways can activate other pro-inflammatory cytokine production, thus generating a vicious circle [43]. Therefore, endothelial dysfunction becomes a promoter of inflammation in the wall vessel and aggravates atherosclerosis [44]. In this metabolic perspective, a sUA level over 8 mg/dL can be considered an indicator of xanthine oxidase activity and an indirect measure of a chronic inflammatory state, much easier to use in clinical practice, compared to cytokine- or endothelial-derived factors [45]. Clinical evaluation of the endothelial function can also be performed by determining circulating levels of markers of endothelial integrity or function, or through functional tests that assess the vascular endothelium in certain areas [46]. Testing the reactivity of the brachial artery with the flow-mediated vasodilatation method has become one of the most used methods, being non-invasive and validated by comparative studies with the standard method [47].

The technique mimics a physiological process of production of NO by activating endothelial NOS parietal response to mechanical stress [48]

SUA level correlates with blood pressure level, with total and visceral adiposity level, with resistance to insulin, fasting glucose level and inversely with triglycerides and HDL-cholesterol levels. Hyperuricemia is an independent predictor for the development of hypertension, diabetes or metabolic syndrome. These correlations are difficult to interpret because of the complex pathogenic relationships between hyperuricemia and hypertension, insulin resistance and kidney disease, but also with oxidative stress metabolism, a crucial mechanism in the cardiovascular pathology [49].

Also, the analysis of the First NHANES Epidemiologic Follow-up Study (NHEFS) found that increased sUA levels were independently and significantly associated with risk of CV mortality among men and women over an average 16.4 year follow-up [50]. Another meta-analysis demonstrates that elevated serum uric acid is associated with a significantly increased risk of suffering from HF [51].

Hyperuricemia may cause or exacerbate ischemic coronary artery disease through the formation of free radicals that leads to decreased bioavailability of nitric oxide with endothelial dysfunction and smooth muscle cell proliferation [40]. Xanthine oxidase activity and uric acid synthesis are increased in vivo under ischemic conditions, and therefore elevated serum uric acid may act as a marker of underlying tissue ischaemia [52]. In the Rotterdam Study the follow-up of 4385 participants over an average of 8.4 years revealed that high sUA levels were a strong predictor of both myocardial infarction and stroke, even after adjusting for other cardiovascular risk factors [4].

A meta-analysis considering studies involving more than 400,000 patients has confirmed the independent association between hyperuricemia and the incidence and mortality from coronary heart disease, with a 12% increase in the overall risk of death for each 1mg/dL of increase in sUA [53].

The prevalence of hyperuricemia is very high in the final stage of the cardiovascular continuum, heart failure. More than 25% of patients with low LVEF have sUA levels> 9.5 mg/dl [54]. In another cross-sectional study, 51% of patients hospitalized for HF had hyperuricemia [55] and sUA levels were higher in cachectic patients with terminal heart failure [56]. Another study determined the level of 8.4 mg/dL for sUA as the cut-off value for increased mortality [57]. There is no general consensus regarding these cut-off values [58]; they range from ≥6.5 mg/dL and 7mg/dL in patients with mild to moderate HF to 8.7 mg/dl and to 9.5 mg/dl in more advanced HF [59].

To test the hypothesis that XO inhibition would improve clinical outcomes in symptomatic HF, the EXACT-HF study randomly assigned 253 high-risk patients with symptomatic left ventricular dysfunction and serum uric acid levels ≥9.5 mg/dL to receive high-dose allopurinol or placebo in a double-blind, multicenter trial. Allopurinol safely lowered uric acid levels in comparison with placebo, but had no detectable benefits on clinical status, exercise capacity, quality of life or left ventricular structure and function. Despite a strong pathophysiological rationale for XO inhibition, positive physiological end points in previous studies may have been poor surrogates for the clinical end points that were measured. Alternatively, this study may have been too short, or the study population too sick to observe a benefit [80]. Also, the mean sUA level was 11 mg/dL and the mean creatinine level 1.5 mg/dL; therefore, hyperuricemia was probably also due to impairment of renal excretion. Filippatos et al. [63] demonstrated the impact of hyperuricemia in patients with HF only when CKD was not associated [60]. The same results were confirmed by a post-hoc analysis of the EVEREST study: hyperuricemia is a predictor for all-cause mortality for patients with eGFR > 30 mL/min/1.73 m^2. In patients with EGFR < 30 ml/min/1.73 m^2, sUA levels have not been correlated with death or rehospitalization of cardiac or non-cardiac causes [76]. Also, other studies proved that if hyperuricemia is caused by impaired renal excretion and not by increased xanthine oxidase activity, the use of xanthine oxidase inhibitors is unlikely to improve outcomes [55, 61, 81].

It remains to be seen, however, if xanthine oxidase inhibitors would improve outcomes in ADHF patients without CKD for whom hyperuricemia is likely caused by increased xanthine oxidase activity and not by impaired renal excretion of uric acid [55].

Elevated sUA levels found in acute heart failure are most likely multifactorial involving besides oxidative metabolism abnormalities [60], impaired kidney function [55, 61], activation of cytokines and insulin resistance [29] Overproduction of sUA is however the dominant factor determining hyperuricemia; due to the increase of the XO substrate [62, 64] (with degradation of ATP to adenosine and hypoxanthine, secondary tissue hypoxia and cell death) and the amplification of the expression and activity of this enzyme. SUA levels in these patients are a witness to the degree of activation of the XO. Experimental evidence demonstrates increased activity of xanthine oxidase in acute heart failure, which causes increased production of superoxide [65]. Through its O2 production, XO may not contribute significantly to ROS production in normal human hearts, but it increases its activity by about 10 fold in ADHF which would increase the relative contribution of this enzyme to oxidative stress [66]. ROS lead to a depression of the excitation-contraction coupling mechanism in cardiac muscle, inducing a decrease in cardiac contractility and in the rate of cardiac muscle relaxation [67].

The sUA level also seems to be a reflection of pulmonary and systemic congestion [58], given the association of hyperuricemia with restrictive pattern of diastolic dysfunction, high filling pressure and right ventricular dysfunction [68, 69] and the close correlation with Killip class in HF in the setting of acute myocardial infarction [70].

NO-dependent regulation of ventricular function and vascular tone determines hemodynamic status in ADHF. Decreased NO availability induces vasoconstriction and increased vascular stiffness in the systemic and pulmonary circulation, resulting in augmented left and right ventricular systolic workload [71]. Decreased NO bioavailability also enhances endothelin-1–induced vasoconstriction, increases sympathetic outflow and catecholamine release and diminishes sodium excretion in the kidney; all these being important in the vicious circle of acute HF syndromes [16].

The angiotensin-converting enzyme has increased activity in ADHF, causing the decrease in the bioavailability of NO in the endothelium [41]. Besides the direct effect of vasoconstriction, Angiotensin II (AT II) has a complex interaction with oxygen free radicals and NO[17]. AT II stimulates superoxide generation by increasing expression NADPH-oxidase gene and its activity. The NO decrease potentiates the vasoconstrictor effect of ATII [22, 23].

As in chronic HF, sUA levels correlate, in acute HF with short and long-term prognosis, uric acid being a witness of the intensification of XO activity, pronounced by secondary tissue hypoxia, inflammation and endothelial and myocyte dysfunction [74]. However, if in CHF the sUA role is better established, being identified some cut-off values for predicting the poor prognosis, in acute HF the prognostic value is not as well known; prospective studies are needed to establish the prognostic value and determine the cutoff levels in this situation. The first attempts showed that high sUA levels were associated with a higher risk of death and new heart failure readmission. Hyperuricemia was also an independent predictor of all-cause mortality in unselected consecutive patients admitted with AHF [31]. Also, Pascual-Figal et al [75] demonstrated that patients hospitalized for decompensated heart failure who had hyperuricemia (defined by the values conventionally used in gout) had an increased risk of mortality and/or cardiac rehospitalization.

A study including 283 patients with ADHF showed that 121 patients (43.1%) had hyperuricemia with mean sUA concentration of 6.4 mg/dL and sUA levels were significantly increased in patients with CKD compared to patients without CKD. However, UA was not associated with the development of acute kidney injury. Elevated sUA levels were associated with both CKD and pulmonary congestion. After controlling for potential confounders, hyperuricemia was associated with rehospitalization and death at 6 months [58]. In conclusion, the prognostic use of sUA differs by baseline renal function, suggesting different biologic and pathophysiologic significance of sUA among those with and without significant renal dysfunction [76].

The Czech national registry AHEAD (Acute Heart Failure Database), that included patients with acute decompensated HF, de novo HF and cardiogenic shock, analyzed 1255 patients who had information on the sUA level at admission. Average sUA concentration was 7.26 mg/dL and higher concentrations than 8.67 mg/dL were associated with increased mortality. Also, a poor correlation was identified between sUA level and NT-proBNP level at admission and discharge. The 1-year survival rate of patients discharged from hospital was 75.6%, and the 2-year rate was 66.8% [57].

Another cohort study with patients of the Japanese Cardiac Registry of Heart Failure (patients hospitalized for decompensated HF) observed the outcomes after discharge of these patients (follow-up period of 2.1 years after discharge). Of the total cohort of HF patients, 56% had hyperuricemia and mean sUA level was 7.3 ± 2.4 mg/dL. Patients with sUA >7.4mg/dL had higher rates of all-cause death, cardiac death and rehospitalization. After multivariable adjustment including eGFR and the use of diuretics, higher sUA level resulted as a significant and independent predictor for all-cause death and cardiac death [77]. There was a 6.8% increase in all-cause death for each 1 mg/dL increase in sUA level. The sUA level was also associated with rehospitalization due to worsening HF [77].

Therefore, elevated sUA levels seem to be a robust and reliable marker of advanced symptomatic state, disease progression and impaired prognosis in ADHF. Assessment of sUA is a simple and non-expensive laboratory measurement that ensures wide clinical availability. It has many of the desired characteristics of an ideal biomarker and should be included of routine assessment in patients with ADHF [76].

Emerging data from clinical studies suggest that XO inhibition could have a role as a tailored treatment option in hyperuricemic patients with ADHF to improve symptomatic status, to attenuate disease progression and potentially improve prognosis [59]. It is tempting to speculate that Allopurinol attenuates ROS-dependent mitochondrial damage and improves diastolic function by improving maximal ADP-stimulated respiratory capacity and ADP/ATP ratio [78, 79]. Also, XO inhibition with Allopurinol improved peripheral blood flow and vasodilatory capacity in hyperuricemic patients [66]. Therefore, the **objectives** of our study were to assess the effect of Allopurinol treatment on endothelial function and sUA levels in ADHF.

Method. Study group included 81 patients hospitalized for ADHF with NYHA class III-IV, caused by ischemic and non-ischemic cardiomyopathy, treated according to 2012 ESH/ESC Guidelines. 42 patients randomly selected (ALLO+) received Allopurinol 300 mg/day regardless of sUA level. sUA and endothelial function were evaluated in all patients at baseline (on admission), on day 2, day 5 and on discharge. Endothelial function was assessed by flow mediated vasodilatation method. Percentage variation in the diameter of brachial artery before and after ischemic stimulus (FMD) was calculated, values below 10% indicating endothelial dysfunction.

Results. Patients included in the study (61% males, mean age 71 ± 10 years) had mean left ventricular ejection fraction (FEVS) of 37 ± 11%. Hyperuricemia (sUA ≥ 7 mg/dL in males and ≥ 6 mg/dL in females) was found in 51% of patients, similar to other studies on ADHF, with the mean sUA at admission of 7.05 ± 2.66 mg/dL. SUA levels significantly decreased in ALLO+ group (Figure 1) and increased in ALLO- group (from 7.44 ± 2.77 mg/dL to 5.21 ± 1.48 mg/dL *vs* 6.63 ± 2.51 mg/dL to 6.98 ± 2.25 mg/dL, $p < 0.001$). The prevalence of hyperuricemia decreased by 76% in ALLO+ and increased by 25% in ALLO- ($p < 0.001$). Mean FMD was 8.46 ± 4.73% at admission vs. 16.26 ± 7.50% at discharge in ALLO+ (Figure 2) and 9.63 ± 8.10% at admission vs. 12.51 ± 8.84% at discharge in ALLO-. Therefore, a significant improvement of endothelial function was observed in ALLO+ group in comparison/compaired to ALLO- group ($p = 0.001$). Endothelial function improved in 29 patients in ALLO+ and in 6 patients in ALLO- ($p < 0.001$).

Our results suggest that in ADHF there is a strong relationship between hyperuricemia and endothelial dysfunction. Allopurinol treatment decreases sUA levels and improves the endothelial function.

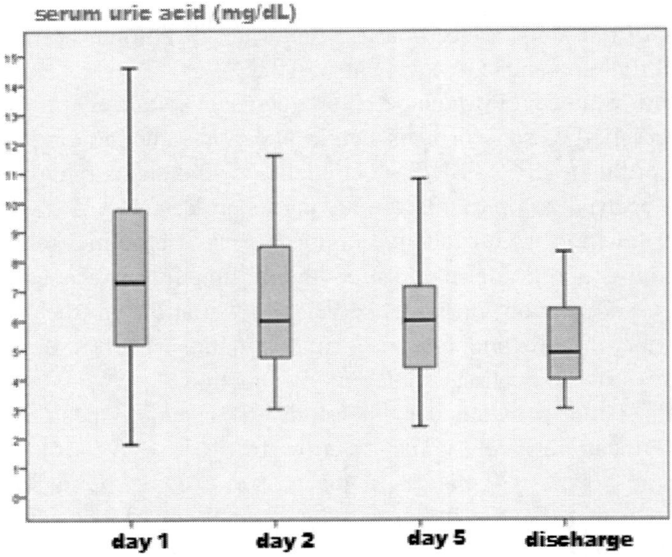

Figure 1. Variation of sUA level (mg/dL) during hospitalization in ALLO+ group.

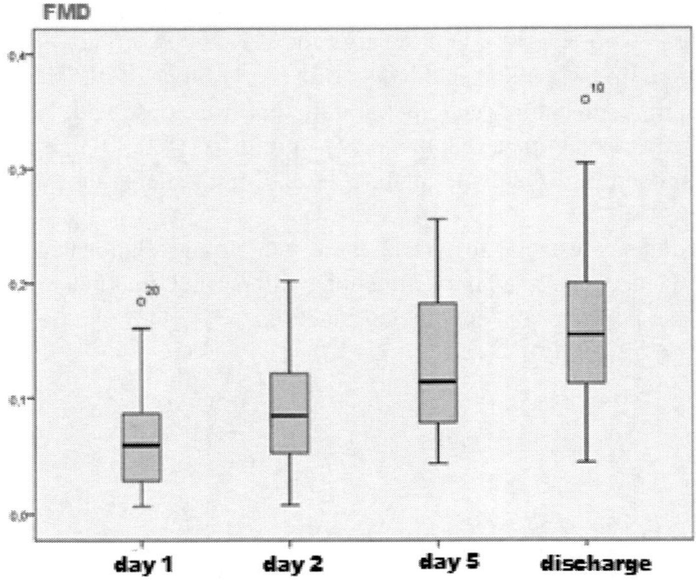

Figure 2. Variation of FMD (%) during hospitalization in ALLO+ group.

References

[1] Dickstein K, Cohen-solal A, Mcmurray JJ V, et al. ESC Guidelines for the diagnosis and treatment of acute and chronic heart failure 2016. *Eur J Heart Fail.* 2016:933-989. doi:10.1016/j.ejheart.2008.08.005.

[2] Mosterd A, Hoes AW, De Bruyne MC, et al. Prevalence of heart failure and left ventricular dysfunction in the general population. The Rotterdam Study. *Eur Heart J.* 1999;20(6):447-455. doi:10.1053/euhj.1998.1239.

[3] Redfield MM, Jacobsen SJ, Burnett JC, Mahoney DW, Bailey KR, Rodeheffer RJ. Burden of Systolic and Diastolic Ventricular. *Intern Med.* 2003;289(2):194-202. doi:10.1001/jama.289.2.194.

[4] Bleumink GS, Knetsch AM, Sturkenboom MCJM, et al. Quantifying the heart failure epidemic: Prevalence, incidence rate, lifetime risk and prognosis of heart failure - The Rotterdam Study. *Eur Heart J.* 2004;25(18):1614-1619. doi:10.1016/j.ehj.2004.06.038.

[5] Ceia F, Fonseca C, Mota T, et al. Prevalence of chronic heart failure in Southwestern Europe: The EPICA study. *Eur J Heart Fail.* 2002;4(4):531-539. doi:10.1016/S1388-9842(02)00034-X.

[6] Stewart S, MacIntyre K, Capewell S, McMurray JJ V. Heart failure and the aging population: an increasing burden in the 21st century? *Heart.* 2003;89(1):49-53. doi:10.1136/heart.89.1.49.

[7] Failure H, States U, Vary HF. Heart Failure Fact Sheet Heart Failure in the United States Deaths from Heart Failure Vary by Geography Risk Factors for Heart Failure Signs and Symptoms of Heart Failure. 2009:2009-2011.

[8] Braunwald E. Heart failure. *JACC Hear Fail.* 2013;1(1):1-20. doi:10.1016/j.jchf.2012.10.002.

[9] McMurray JJ V, Adamopoulos S, Anker SD, et al. ESC Guidelines for the diagnosis and treatment of acute and chronic heart failure 2012: The Task Force for the Diagnosis and Treatment of Acute and Chronic Heart Failure 2012 of the European Society of Cardiology. Developed in collaboration with the Heart. *Rev Port Cardiol.* 2013;32(7-8):e1-e641 - e61. doi:10.1093/eurheartj/ehs104.

[10] Wang TJ, Evans JC, Benjamin EJ, Levy D, LeRoy EC, Vasan RS. Natural history of asymptomatic left ventricular systolic dysfunction in the community. *Circulation.* 2003;108(8):977-982. doi:10.1161/01.CIR.0000085166.44904.79.

[11] Heidenreich PA, Trogdon JG, Khavjou OA, et al. Forecasting the future of cardiovascular disease in the United States: A policy statement from the American Heart Association. *Circulation*. 2011;123(8):933-944. doi:10.1161/CIR.0b013e31820a55f5.

[12] Go AS, Mozaffarian D, Roger VL, et al. Heart disease and stroke statistics-2013 update: A Report from the American Heart Association. *Circulation*. 2013;127(1). doi:10.1161/CIR.0b013e31828124ad.

[13] Van Riet EES, Hoes AW, Limburg A, Landman MAJ, Van Der Hoeven H, Rutten FH. Prevalence of unrecognized heart failure in older persons with shortness of breath on exertion. *Eur J Heart Fail*. 2014;16(7):772-777. doi:10.1002/ejhf.110.

[14] Marti CN, Gheorghiade M, Kalogeropoulos AP, Georgiopoulou V V, Quyyumi AA, Butler J. Endothelial dysfunction, arterial stiffness, and heart failure. *J Am Coll Cardiol*. 2012;60(16):1455-1469. doi:10.1016/j.jacc.2011.11.082.

[15] Ho KKL, Pinsky JL, Kannel WB, Levy D. The epidemiology of heart failure: The Framingham Study. *J Am Coll Cardiol*. 1993;22(4 SUPPL. 1). doi:10.1016/0735-1097(93)90455-A.

[16] Maggioni AP, Dahlstr??m U, Filippatos G, et al. EURObservational research programme: The heart failure Pilot survey (ESC-HF Pilot). *Eur J Heart Fail*. 2010;12(10):1076-1084. doi:10.1093/eurjhf/hfq154.

[17] Pocock SJ, Ariti CA, McMurray JJ V, et al. Predicting survival in heart failure: A risk score based on 39 372 patients from 30 studies. *Eur Heart J*. 2013;34(19):1404-1413. doi:10.1093/eurheartj/ehs337.

[18] Chen J, Normand S-LT, Wang Y, Krumholz HM. National and regional trends in heart failure hospitalization and mortality rates for Medicare beneficiaries, 1998-2008. *Jama*. 2011;306(15):1669-1678. doi:10.1001/jama.2011.1474.

[19] Kochanek KD, Xu J, Murphy SL, H AMMMP. Deaths : Preliminary Data for 2009. *Natl Vital Stat Reports*. 2011;59(4):1-51. doi:http://198.246.98.21/nchs/data/nvsr/nvsr59/nvsr59_04.pdf.

[20] Moser DK, Mann DL. Improving outcomes in heart failure: It's not unusual beyond usual care. *Circulation*. 2002;105(24):2810-2812. doi:10.1161/01.CIR.0000021745.45349.BB.

[21] Daniel I. Feig, Duk-Hee Kang, Johnson RJ. Uric Acid and Cardiovasclar Risk. *N Engl J Med*. 2009;359(17):1811-1821. doi:10.1056/NEJMra0800885.Uric.

[22] Johnson RJ, Sautin YY, Oliver WJ, et al. NIH Public Access. *J Comp Physiol*. 2009;179(1):67-76. doi:10.1007/s00360-008-0291-7.Lessons.

[23] Desideri G, Castaldo G, Lombardi A, et al. Is it time to revise the normal range of serum uric acid levels? *Eur Rev Med Pharmacol Sci*. 2014;18(9):1295-1306.

[24] Berry CE, Hare JM. Xanthine oxidoreductase and cardiovascular disease: molecular mechanisms and pathophysiological implications. *J Physiol*. 2004;555(Pt 3):589-606. doi:10.1113/jphysiol.2003.055913.

[25] Puddu P, Puddu GM, Cravero E, Vizioli L, Muscari A. The relationships among hyperuricemia, endothelial dysfunction, and cardiovascular diseases: Molecular mechanisms and clinical implications. *J Cardiol*. 2012;59(3):235-242. doi:10.1016/j.jjcc.2012.01.013.

[26] Lippi G, Montagnana M, Franchini M, Favaloro EJ, Targher G. The paradoxical relationship between serum uric acid and cardiovascular disease. *Clin Chim Acta*. 2008;392(1-2):1-7. doi:10.1016/j.cca.2008.02.024.

[27] Leyva F, Anker S, Swan JW, et al. Serum uric acid as an index of impaired oxidative metabolism in chronic heart failure. *Eur Heart J*. 1997;18:858-865.

[28] Bagnati M, Perugini C, Cau C, Bordone R, Albano E, Bellomo G. When and why a water-soluble antioxidant becomes pro-oxidant during copper-induced low-density lipoprotein oxidation: a study using uric acid. *Biochem J*. 1999;340 (Pt 1:143-152. doi:10.1042/0264-6021:3400143.

[29] Iliesiu A, Campeanu A, Dusceac D. Serum uric acid and cardiovascular disease. *M{æ}dica*. 2010;5(3):186-192. http://www.ncbi.nlm.nih.gov/pubmed/23352265.

[30] Khan SA, Lee K, Minhas KM, et al. Neuronal nitric oxide synthase negatively regulates xanthine oxidoreductase inhibition of cardiac excitation-contraction coupling. *Proc Natl Acad Sci U S A*. 2004;101(45):15944-15948. doi:10.1073/pnas.0404136101.

[31] Mazzali M, Hughes J, Kim YG, et al. Elevated uric acid increases blood pressure in the rat by a novel crystal-independent mechanism. *Hypertension*. 2001;38(5):1101-1106. doi:10.1161/hy1101.092839.

[32] Higgins P, Dawson J, Walters M. The potential for xanthine oxidase inhibition in the prevention and treatment of cardiovascular and cerebrovascular disease. *Cardiovasc Psychiatry Neurol*. 2009; 2009:282059. doi:10.1155/2009/282059.

[33] Bickel C, Rupprecht HJ, Blankenberg S, et al. Serum uric acid as an independent predictor of mortality in patients with angiographically proven coronary artery disease. *Am J Cardiol.* 2002;89(1):12-17. doi:10.1016/S0002-9149(01)02155-5.

[34] Hadi HAR, Carr CS, Al Suwaidi J. Endothelial dysfunction: cardiovascular risk factors, therapy, and outcome. *Vasc Health Risk Manag*. 2005;1(3):183-198. doi:10.1016/j.diabres.2008.12.013.

[35] Perticone F, Ceravolo R, Pujia A. Prognostic significance of endothelial dysfunction in hypertensive patients. *Circulation.* 2001. http://circ.ahajournals.org/content/104/2/191.short.

[36] Yamamoto E, Hirata Y, Tokitsu T, et al. The pivotal role of eNOS uncoupling in vascular endothelial dysfunction in patients with heart failure with preserved ejection fraction. *Int J Cardiol.* 2015;190(1):335-337. doi:10.1016/j.ijcard.2015.04.162.

[37] Khosla UM, Zharikov S, Finch JL, et al. Hyperuricemia induces endothelial dysfunction. *Kidney Int.* 2005;67(5):1739-1742. doi:10.1111/j.1523-1755.2005.00273.x.

[38] Shimbo D, Grahame-Clarke C, Miyake Y, et al. The association between endothelial dysfunction and cardiovascular outcomes in a population-based multi-ethnic cohort. *Atherosclerosis.* 2007;192(1):197-203. doi:10.1016/j.atherosclerosis.2006.05.005.

[39] Karantalis V, Schulman IH, Hare JM. Nitroso-redox imbalance affects cardiac structure and function. *J Am Coll Cardiol.* 2013;61(9):933-935. doi:10.1016/j.jacc.2012.12.016.

[40] et al. Costa, Sonia; Reina-Couto, Marta; Albino-Texeira A. Statins and oxidative stress in chronic heart failure. *Rev Port Cardiol.* 2016;36(1):41-57. doi:10.1016/j.repce.2015.12.016.

[41] Ruggiero C, Cherubini A, Ble A, et al. Uric acid and inflammatory markers. *Eur Heart J.* 2006;27(10):1174-1181. doi:10.1093/eurheartj/ehi879.

[42] De Caterina R, Libby P, Peng HB, et al. Nitric oxide decreases cytokine-induced endothelial activation: Nitric oxide selectively reduces endothelial expression of adhesion molecules and proinflammatory cytokines. *J Clin Invest.* 1995;96(1):60-68. doi:10.1172/JCI118074.

[43] Baldasseroni S, Urso R, Maggioni a P, et al. Prognostic significance of serum uric acid in outpatients with chronic heart failure is complex and related to body mass index: data from the IN-CHF Registry. *Nutr Metab Cardiovasc Dis.* 2012;22(5):442-448. doi:10.1016/j.numecd.2010.08.007.

[44] Benjamin EJ, Larson MG, Keyes MJ, et al. Clinical Correlates and Heritability of Flow-Mediated Dilation in the Community: The Framingham Heart Study. *Circulation.* 2004;109(5):613-619. doi:10.1161/01.CIR.0000112565.60887.1E.

[45] Corretti MC, Anderson TJ, Benjamin EJ, et al. Guidelines for the ultrasound assessment of endothelial-dependent flow- mediated vasodilation of the brachial artery: a report of the International Brachial Artery Reactivity Task Force. *J Am Coll Cardiol.* 2002;39(2):257-265.

[46] McMackin CJ, Vita JA. Update on nitric oxide-dependent vasodilation in human subjects. *Methods Enzymol.* 2005;396(05):541-553. doi:10.1016/S0076-6879(05)96046-1.

[47] Tae WY, Ki CS, Hun SS, Col. Relationship between serum uric acid concentration and insulin resistance and metabolic syndrome. *Circ J.* 2005;69(8):928-933. doi:10.1253/circj.69.928.

[48] Wu AH, Gladden JD, Ahmed M, Ahmed A, Filippatos G. Relation of serum uric acid to cardiovascular disease. *Int J Cardiol.* 2015:8-11. doi:10.1016/j.ijcard.2015.08.110.

[49] Huang H, Huang B, Li Y, et al. Uric acid and risk of heart failure: A systematic review and meta-analysis. *Eur J Heart Fail.* 2014;16(1):15-24. doi:10.1093/eurjhf/hft132.

[50] Fang J, Alderman MH. Serum Uric Acid and Cardiovascular Mortality. *Jama.* 2000;283(5):2404. doi:10.1001/jama.283.18.2404.

[51] Volterrani M, Iellamo F, Sposato B, Romeo F. Uric acid lowering therapy in cardiovascular diseases. *Int J Cardiol.* 2015:8-10. doi:10.1016/j.ijcard.2015.08.088.

[52] Kittleson MM, St John ME, Bead V, et al. Increased levels of uric acid predict haemodynamic compromise in patients with heart failure independently of B-type natriuretic peptide levels. *Heart.* 2007;93(3):365-367. doi:10.1136/hrt.2006.090845.

[53] Ekundayo OJ, Dell'Italia LJ, Sanders PW, et al. Association between hyperuricemia and incident heart failure among older adults: A propensity-matched study. *Int J Cardiol.* 2010;142(3):279-287. doi:10.1016/j.ijcard.2009.01.010.

[54] Anker SD, Doehner W, Rauchhaus M, et al. Uric acid and survival in chronic heart: Failure validation and application in metabolic, functional, and hemodynamic staging. *Circulation.* 2003;107(15):1991-1997. doi:10.1161/01.CIR.0000065637.10517.A0.

[55] Málek F, Ošťádal P, Pařenica J, et al. Uric acid, allopurinol therapy, and mortality in patients with acute heart failure-results of the Acute HEart FAilure Database registry. *J Crit Care*. 2012;27(6). doi:10.1016/j.jcrc.2012.03.011.

[56] Palazzuoli A, Ruocco G, Pellegrini M, et al. Prognostic Significance of Hyperuricemia in Patients with Acute Heart Failure. *Am J Cardiol*. 2016:1-6. doi:10.1016/j.amjcard. 2016.02.039.

[57] Doehner W, Jankowska EA, Springer J, Lainscak M, Anker SD. Uric acid and xanthine oxidase in heart failure — Emerging data and therapeutic implications. *Int J Cardiol*. 2015. doi:10.1016/ j.ijcard.2015.08.089.

[58] Patel P, Arora R. Uric acid and xanthine oxidase: perspectives in chronic heart failure. *Arch Med Sci*. 2008;4(3):219-225. http://www.termedia.pl/Czasopismo/Archives{_}of{_} Medical{_}Science-19/Artykul-11189.

[59] Repository ZO. University of Zurich Uric acid in chronic heart failure - current pathophysiological concepts. 2008;10(12):1269-1270.

[60] Doehner W, von Haehling S, Anker SD. Uric acid as a prognostic marker in acute heart failure--new expectations from an old molecule. *Eur J Hear Fail J Work Gr Hear Fail Eur Soc Cardiol*. 2007;9(5):437-439. doi:10.1016/j.ejheart.2007.03.006.

[61] Filippatos GS, Ahmed MI, Gladden JD, et al. Hyperuricaemia, chronic kidney disease, and outcomes in heart failure: Potential mechanistic insights from epidemiological data. *Eur Heart J*. 2011;32(6):712-720. doi:10.1093/eurheartj/ehq473.

[62] Doehner W, von Haehling S, Anker SD. Uric acid in CHF: Marker or player in a metabolic disease? *Int J Cardiol*. 2007;115(2):156-158. doi:10.1016/j.ijcard.2006.05.003.

[63] Bergamini C, Cicoira M, Rossi A, Vassanelli C. Oxidative stress and hyperuricaemia: Pathophysiology, clinical relevance, and therapeutic implications in chronic heart failure. *Eur J Heart Fail*. 2009;11(5):444-452. doi:10.1093/eurjhf/hfp042.

[64] Cingolani HE, Plastino JA, Escudero EM, Mangal B, Brown J, P??rez NG. The Effect of Xanthine Oxidase Inhibition Upon Ejection Fraction in Heart Failure Patients: La Plata Study. *J Card Fail*. 2006;12(7):491-498. doi:10.1016/j.cardfail.2006.05.005.

[65] Radovanovic S, Savic-Radojevic A, Pekmezovic T, et al. Uric acid and gamma-glutamyl transferase activity are associated with left ventricular remodeling indices in patients with chronic heart failure. *Rev espa{ñ}ola Cardiol (English ed)*. 2014;67(8):632-642. doi:10.1016/j.rec.2013.11.017.

[66] Chrysohoou C, Pitsavos C, Barbetseas J, et al. Serum uric acid levels correlate with left atrial function and systolic right ventricular function in patients with newly diagnosed heart failure: the hellenic heart failure study. *Congest Hear Fail*. 2008;14(october):229-233. doi:10.1111/j.1751-7133.2008.00005.x.

[67] Amin A, Vakilian F, Maleki M. Serum uric acid levels correlate with filling pressures in systolic heart failure. *Congest Heart Fail*. 2011;17(2):80-84. doi:10.1111/j.1751-7133.2010.00205.x.

[68] Alimonda AL, Nunez J, Nunez E, et al. Hyperuricemia in acute heart failure. More than a simple spectator? *Eur J Intern Med*. 2009;20(1):74-79. doi:10.1016/j.ejim.2008.04.007.

[69] Iliesiu A, Campeanu A, Marta D, Parvu I. Uric Acid, Oxidative Stress and Inflammation in Chronic Heart Failure with Reduced Ejection Fraction. *Rev Rom Med Lab*. 2015;23(4):397-406. doi:10.1515/rrlm-2015-0039.

[70] Heart IJC, Yamamoto E, Ohba K, et al. Olmesartan reverses not only vascular endothelial dysfunction but cardiac diastolic dysfunction in hypertensive patients with heart failure with preserved ejection fraction — ORION study. *IJCHA*. 2015;8:128-130. doi:10.1016/j.ijcha.2015.06.002.

[71] Widlansky ME, Gokce N, Keaney JF, Vita JA. The clinical implications of endothelial dysfunction. *J Am Coll Cardiol*. 2003;42(7):1149-1160. doi:10.1016/S0735-1097(03)00
994-X.

[72] Kurata A, Shigematsu Y, Higaki J. Sex-Related Differences in Relations of Uric Acid to Left Ventricular Hypertrophy and Remodeling in Japanese Hypertensive Patients. 2005;28(2):133-139. doi:10.1291/hypres.28.133.

[73] Pascual-Figal DA, Hurtado-Martínez JA, Redondo B, Antolinos MJ, Ruiperez JA, Valdes M. Hyperuricaemia and long-term outcome after hospital discharge in acute heart failure patients. *Eur J Heart Fail*. 2007;9(5):518-524. doi:10.1016/j.ejheart.2006.09.001.

[74] Vaduganathan M, Greene SJ, Ambrosy AP, et al. Relation of serum uric acid levels and outcomes among patients hospitalized for worsening heart failure with reduced ejection fraction (from the efficacy of vasopressin antagonism in heart failure outcome study with tolvaptan trial). *Am J Cardiol.* 2014;114(11):1713-1721. doi:10.1016/j.amjcard.2014.09.008.

[75] Hamaguchi S, Furumoto T, Tsuchihashi-Makaya M, et al. Hyperuricemia predicts adverse outcomes in patients with heart failure. *Int J Cardiol.* 2011;151(2):143-147. doi:10.1016/j.ijcard.2010.05.002.

[76] Ekelund UE, Harrison RW, Shokek O, et al. Intravenous allopurinol decreases myocardial oxygen consumption and increases mechanical efficiency in dogs with pacing-induced heart failure. *Circ Res.* 1999;85(5):437-445. doi:10.1161/01.RES.85.5.437.

[77] Cappola TP, Kass DA, Nelson GS, et al. Allopurinol improves myocardial efficiency in patients with idiopathic dilated cardiomyopathy. *Circulation.* 2001;104(20):2407-2411. doi:10.1161/hc4501.098928.

[78] Bellomo G. The relationship between uric acid, allopurinol, cardiovascular events, and kidney disease progression: A step forward. *Am J Kidney Dis.* 2015;65(4):525-527. doi:10.1053/j.ajkd.2015.01.001.

[79] Gavin a D, Struthers a D. Allopurinol reduces B-type natriuretic peptide concentrations and haemoglobin but does not alter exercise capacity in chronic heart failure. *Heart.* 2005;91(6):749-753. doi:10.1136/hrt.2004.040477.

BIOGRAPHICAL SKETCH

Alexandru CAMPEANU

Affiliation: Professor of Internal Medicine and Cardiology with the "Carol Davila" University of Medicine and Pharmacy, Bucharest; "Prof. Dr. Th. Burghele" Clinical Hospital, Department of Internal Medicine and Cardiology, Bucharest

Education: Senior Cardiologist and Internist, PhD in Medical Sciences, habilitation in electrocardiography and echocardiography, participant in excellence courses on a national and international level.

Research and Professional Experience:

Professional experience:

-2000 – Present: Professor of Internal Medicine and Cardiology with the "Carol Davila" University of Medicine and Pharmacy, Bucharest; "Prof. Dr. Th. Burghele" Clinical Hospital, Department of Internal Medicine and Cardiology, Bucharest. PhD advisor. Director of teaching courses, workshops.

-1974 – 2000: Lecturer with the "Carol Davila" University of Medicine and Pharmacy, Bucharest;

-1964 – 1974: Assistant Professor with the "Carol Davila" University of Medicine and Pharmacy, Bucharest.

Research projects:

Participation in International and National Trials: SYMPHONY, CITAS, HERO, EPHESUS, PARSIFAL, AMISTAD, APRES

Member of Steering Committee and National Coordinator of EPHESUS and CITAS Trials

Scientific Coordinator of ALO-HF Studies Project CNCSIS-UEFISCSU IDEI no. 1451/2008. Title: Effects Of Allopurinol On Oxidative Stress, Serum Uric Acid, Cardiac Function And Remodeling In Patients With Chronic Heart Failure. Acronym: ALLO-HF. Period: 2008-2011

Professional Appointments:

Member of the Romanian Academy of Medical Sciences;

Member of Heart Failure Working Group of the European Society of Cardiology;

Member of the Federation of Heart Failure, European Society of Cardiology;

Member of the International Society Cardiovascular Pharmacotherapy;

Member of the editorial board of Romanian Journal of Cardiology Bucharest.

Honors

-1973 – PhD with the thesis "Studies Concerning Etiology of Acute Pneumonias – Role of Viruses and Mixed Infections; Epidemiology and Diagnosis of Pneumonias"

-Member of the Romanian Academy of Medical Sciences

-Invited conferences during numerous international and national scientific events, chairperson during international and national scientific events

International distinctions:

1. Effects of High Dose Allopurinol on Clinical Outcome,Cardiac Function, Quality of Life and Effort Capacity in Patients with Symptomatic Chronic Heart Failure. AM. Iliesiu; **AL. Campeanu**; D.Dusceac; A. Cristea; G. Uscoiu; T. Nanea. "Heart Failure 2013" Lisbon-Portugal, 25-28 May 2013. P1128. European Journal of Heart Failure Supplements (2013) 12, S73–S325; doi:10.1093/eurjhf/hst009 – Selected for the Clinical highlights of the Heart Failure 2013 Congress
2. Left atrial mechanical function in hypertensive patients. A Iliesiu, Irina Andrei, Camelia Nicolae,N. Paun, Brandusa Strejan, **A. Campeanu**, T. Nanea. X World Congress of Echocardiography and Cardiovascular Imaging, Roma 19-21 Oct, 2006 – 3rd Prize in the Poster Section

The scientific activity includes more than 200 papers published in journals, books and Congress Proceedings.

In: Uric Acid
Editor: Mary Newman

ISBN: 978-1-53610-287-1

Chapter 4

EFFECT OF ALLOPURINOL ON SERUM URIC ACID, ENDOTHELIAL FUNCTION AND PLATELET AGGREGATION IN PATIENTS WITH ARTERIAL HYPERTENSION

Andreea Simona Hodorogea[1]*, MD, PhD,
Alexandru Câmpeanu[1], MD, PhD,
Adriana Mihaela Ilieșiu[1], MD, PhD,
Gabriela Silvia Gheorghe[1], MD, PhD,
Valentina Uscătescu[2], MD, PhD
Irina Pârvu[1]
and Ioan Tiberiu Nanea[1], MD, PhD

[1]Department of Internal Medicine and Cardiology,
"Carol Davila" University of Medicine and Pharmacy,
"Theodor Burghele" Clinical Hospital, Bucharest, Romania
[2]Fundeni Clinical Institute, Bucharest, Romania

---

* Corresponding Author: andreea.hodorogea@gmail.com.

ABSTRACT

Allopurinol, a xanthine oxidase inhibitor, has significant evidence of beneficial effect in cardiovascular disease. However, there are conflicting data related to the efficacy of allopurinol treatment in arterial hypertension. The purpose of the study was the assessment of allopurinol effects on endothelial and platelet function in patients with controlled essential arterial hypertension.

Seventy six of one hundred thirty nine optimally treated hypertensive patients were randomly assigned to receive allopurinol 300 mg/day, regardless of serum uric acid level. Serum uric acid level, endothelial function (assessed by flow-mediated vasodilatation) and platelet aggregation response to adenosine diphosphate and collagen (by optical aggregometry method) were determined at baseline and after one month. Endothelial function was also reassessed after 3 and 6 months.

After allopurinol treatment, serum uric acid level significantly and persistently decreased, irrespective of the baseline level. In patients with allopurinol treatment blood pressure was slightly, but significantly lower. The endothelial function improved with allopurinol, more significantly in patients with higher cardiovascular risk. Allopurinol significantly decreased platelet aggregation to adenosine diphosphate and collagen, regardless of concomitant treatment with aspirin.

In conclusion, allopurinol could be an useful complementary treatment in arterial hypertension, having beneficial effects on endothelial and platelet function, essential pathogenic mechanisms in cardiovascular disease.

INTRODUCTION

The association between serum uric acid (sUA) and arterial hypertension (HT) was mentioned as early as 1879, in the first paper on essential HT [1]. Subsequently numerous epidemiological studies have confirmed the correlation between elevated sUA and cardiovascular risk factors, cardiovascular complications and cardiovascular risk [2, 3, 4, 5, 6]. Experimental studies have shown the pathogenic involvement of uric acid in the development of HT and cardiovascular disease progression [7, 8, 9]. The connecting link is oxidative stress, which is one of the pathophysiologic substrates throughout the "cardiovascular continuum," leading to the progression from risk factors to target organ damage and cardiovascular events [10, 11, 12]. Serum uric acid is the end product of purine metabolism. Together with oxygen free radicals, it is the result of the xanthine oxidase enzyme, an important source of oxidative stress [13, 14]. Meanwhile, sUA is the most important endogenous antioxidant, defining "uric acid paradox" [13]. Increased levels of sUA in patients with cardiovascular pathology could be a witness of growing oxidative stress or an attempt to compensate prooxidant status by production of a powerful antioxidant, without involving a direct prooxidant effect of this molecule [13].

Xanthine oxidase inhibitor allopurinol showed significant benefits in cardiovascular disease, largely attributed to blocking a major source of free radicals and also decreasing sUA level. Important evidence proves that the cardiovascular effects of allopurinol are due to endothelial dysfunction improvement, which has been demonstrated in patients with cardiovascular risk factors or cardiovascular pathology (smokers, patients with HT, metabolic syndrome, diabetes, sleep apnea, chronic kidney disease, ischemic heart disease and heart failure) [15, 16, 17, 18, 19, 20, 21, 22, 23, 24, 25, 26, 27, 28, 29, 30, 31]. Improvement of endothelial dysfunction could explain the blood pressure (BP) lowering effect of allopurinol [32, 33, 34]. However, the effect of allopurinol in patients with controlled HT has not been studied yet.

Oxidative stress and activation of inflammation, involved directly or through endothelial dysfunction in coagulation and fibrinolysis pathways or platelet changes, explains pro thrombotic and pro atherogenic status of HT, essential in target organ damage progression and cardiovascular events production [35, 36]. Although it has been shown that allopurinol improves endothelial dysfunction by reducing the vascular oxidative stress, a possible effect (directly or by oxidative stress pathways) on platelet function has not been studied [37, 38, 39, 40, 41]. There is also evidence on the direct involvement of uric acid in the thrombotic process, suggesting a possible beneficial effect of allopurinol through this link [42].

Purpose

The aims of the study were to assess the effect of allopurinol on endothelial and platelet function in patients with essential HT with optimal therapeutic control, in relation to its effect of lowering sUA and to the severity of HT.

METHOD

Study group consisted of 151 patients with essential HT optimally treated as recommended by the 2013 European Society of Cardiology Guidelines [43] Secondary HT, uncontrolled high BP values (over 140/90 in two consecutive measurements), secondary causes of hyperuricemia: decreased renal excretion of sUA (renal impairment with glomerular filtration rate below 30 mL/min/1.73 m^2, hyperparathyroidism, hypothyroidism), increased production of sUA by increased cell turnover or by medication, chronic treatment with allopurinol or known intolerance to allopurinol, concomitant medication with uricosuric agents, severe comorbidities, (decompensated heart failure, acute coronary syndromes, acute respiratory failure, liver cirrhosis, unbalanced diabetes, acute infection), abnormal platelet number or function, intracardiac metal devices or metallic cardiac valves were exclusion criteria [43]. Patients were included in the study after signing the informed consent form, designed in accordance with the Declaration of Helsinki and approved by the Ethics Committee of the Hospital.

All patients included in the study were evaluated for initial diagnosis and staging of HT, according to the ESC Guidelines [43]. In all patients there were performed: history, physical examination, laboratory routine testing (hematology, biochemistry, urine analysis), electrocardiogram (ECG), transthoracic echocardiography, abdominal ultrasound, vascular ultrasound of neck artery, ankle-brachial index, automatic ambulatory BP monitoring for 24 hours (ABPM). The initial assessment was meant to establish the complete diagnosis of HT, to detect associated risk factors, clinical or subclinical target organ damage and to objectify optimal BP control. Based on the degree of HT (1, 2 or 3), the number of risk factors, subclinical organ damage, symptomatic cardiovascular disease, presence of diabetes mellitus and chronic kidney disease, each patient was allocated to one of the 10 years cardiovascular death risk categories (low, moderate, high or very high), as recommended by the ESC Guidelines [43]. At the initial evaluation, all patients were evaluated for sUA levels, endothelial function (evaluated by flow-mediated vasodilation of the brachial artery method) and platelet function (assessed by optical aggregometry method).

The Study Protocol

After the initial assessment, all patients (n=151) continued their previous treatment regimen. 76 of them were randomly assigned (1:1 randomization) to receive allopurinol 300 mg/day, regardless of the sUA level, constituting ALLO + group. The other 75 patients constituted ALLO- group:

Endothelial function was assessed by flow-mediated vasodilation of the brachial artery (FMD) method, as recommended by international guidelines on patient preparation, measurement technique and results reporting [44, 45, 46]. Measurements were performed in the early morning, in a quiet room with controlled temperature (22-25°C) by two experienced observers who were unaware of the patient's treatment scheme. Patients were evaluated supine after at least 10 minutes rest. Tensiometer cuff was positioned 5 cm above the elbow. A linear transducer with a frequency of 10 MHz of Prosound SSD-4000 ultrasound machine (Aloka Co. Ltd) with availability of concomitant pulsed and color Doppler registration was used. Measurements were ECG guided. Brachial artery was identified at the elbow using color Doppler flow. For the measurement of the diameters a longitudinal 2D section of the brachial artery was used in the best image that could identify the arterial lumen, with the intima-lumen interface clearly visible on both the front and the posterior wall. A complete cardiac cycle was recorded and the initial diameter (Di) of the brachial artery was determined as the average of the diastolic (R-wave peak) and systolic (top of the T wave) measured diameters. Ischemic stimulus was created by inflating the cuff to 50 mmHg above the systolic BP. Cuff pressure was kept constant for 5 minutes. 30 seconds after cuff deflation, two-dimensional image of the brachial artery in the same section was registered continuously for 90 seconds, tracking the maximum diameter, which was considered the final diameter (Df). The end result was reported as the percentage change in the diameter of the brachial artery before and after ischemic stimulation: $FMD\% = (Df - Di) x 100 / Di$. The value of 10% was considered as the reference percentage of maximum dilatation of brachial artery after ischemic stimulus removal [47]. Endothelial dysfunction can be identified by FMD values below 10% [47, 48].

Platelet function was assessed by optical aggregometry method in the Hemostasis and Fibrinolysis Laboratory of the Fundeni Clinical Institute, respecting standardization recommendations [49, 50, 51, 52, 53]. Blood samples used for platelet function analysis were collected fasting, from a superficial vein of the upper limb with a 21-gauge needle gauge using a tourniquet that was removed immediately after insertion of the needle into the vein. Venous blood was collected in sealed plastic tubes (two tubes for each patient) containing anticoagulant citrate 3.2% / 0.109 M in a ratio of 1: 9 (1 part anticoagulant to 9 parts blood), transported and stored at room temperature (20- 25°C) and then processed at least 30 minutes and up to 4 hours after collection, by an experienced technician. Each tube was centrifuged separately at room temperature: platelet-rich plasma (PRP) was prepared by centrifugation at 200 x g for 10 minutes and the platelet-poor plasma (PPP) by centrifugation at 1500 x g for 15 minutes. 135 μL of plasma from each tube was transferred to silicone glass containers, which were placed inside the analyzer (Whole Blood Lumi Aggregometer 560C (Chrono Log Corporation, Havertown, PA, USA)) and pre-incubated for 5 minutes at 37°C. In the container with PRP 15 μL of an agonist of platelet aggregation was added, together with a fine piece of iron used to mix the agonist with plasma in a magnetic field within the device. In all patients platelet function was evaluated using as agonists adenosine 5 diphosphate (ADP) 5μM and collagen 3 μg/mL. For each agonist analysis was done independently. Inside the analyzer plasma containers (PRP + agonist or PPP) are located between a monochromatic light beam (620 nm) and a photoelectric cell and the formation of platelet aggregates is detected by analyzing the changing in light transmission (optical density). Initially PRP has high optical density and light is not transmitted at all (0%) but PPP has small optical density and the light beam is fully transmitted (100%). After the addition of an agonist platelets aggregate and absorb less light so that the light transmission progressively increases from 0 to 100%. Recording was done for 5 minutes. The maximum response was noted (maximum aggregation) which was expressed as a percentage and was calculated by the formula: *maximum aggregation (%) = [(0% aggregation (PRP initial) – 100% aggregation (PPP initial))/ maximum aggregation] x 100.*

Statistical analysis was performed using Statistica 8.0. Quantitative variables were shown by mean and standard deviation. For comparison between variables $\chi 2$ and Fisher exact tests (dichotomous variables), Mann-Whitney and Wilcoxon tests (ordinal and quantitative variables with non-normal distribution), Student (t) test (quantitative variables with normal distribution) were used. For correlation analysis within the same group of variables Spearman coefficient Kendall test (ordinal and quantitative variables with non-normal distribution) or linear regression and Pearson correlation coefficient (r) (quantitative variables with normal distribution) were used. The statistical significance threshold was chosen for p-values <0.05 and $r> 0.25$.

RESULTS

Of the 76 patients initially included in ALLO + 7 have voluntarily waived and 2 were lost to follow, so only 67 patients presented at the assessment at 6 months. Of the 75 patients initially included in ALLO- one patient voluntarily withdrew to participate in the study in the first month, 2 were lost to follow, and the remaining 72 patients presented for reevaluation at 3 and 6 months. The final study group (n = 139) consisted of 67 patients in ALLO+ and 72 patients in ALLO-.

The characteristics of the two groups of patients at baseline are presented in Table 1. The results show the homogeneity of the groups, with no significant differences between the analyzed parameters.

Table 1. Baseline characteristics of the study group

Baseline characteristics	Total (n=139)	ALLO + (n = 67)	ALLO- (n = 72)	p (ALLO+/ ALLO-)
Demographics				
Age (years)	60.33 ± 12.03	61.81 ± 10.67	59.4 ± 12.83	0.29
Gender (F/M)- n(%)	69 (49.6)/70(50.4)	28 (41.8)/39(58.2)	41(56.9)/ 31 (43.06)	0.014
HT grade				0.35
Grade 1- n(%)	11 (7.9)	3 (4.5)	8 (11.1)	
Grade 2- n(%)	39 (28.1)	21 (31.3)	18 (25)	
Grade 3 - n(%)	89 (64.0)	43 (64.2)	46 (63.9)	
Average SBP/24 h (mmHg) ABPM	140.95 ± 14.16	139.96 ± 14.94	142.76 ± 13.26	0.16
Average DBP/24 h(mmHg) ABPM	86.69 ± 13.92	84.99 ± 13.09	88.25 ± 14.57	0.22
Cardiovascular risk factors				
Family medical history - n(%)	51 (36.7)	24 (35.8)	27 (37.5)	0.39
Smoking - n(%)	46 (33.1)	28 (41.8)	18 (25.0)	0.045
Hypercholesterolemia - n(%)	111 (79.9)	53 (79.1)	58 (80.6)	0.81
Abdominal obesity	111 (79.9)	55 (82.1)	56 (77.8)	0.33
Waist circumference (cm)	100.96 ±13.71	104.37 ±15.39	98.73±12.09	0.03
Obesity (IMC > 30 kg/mp)	58 (41.7)	26 (38.8)	32 (44.40)	0.67
BMI (kg/m^2)	28.90±5.59	29.37±6.67	28.58±4.8	0.44
Prediabetes- n(%)	42 (30.2)	18 (26.9)	24 (33.3)	0.53
Subclinical organ damage				
Renal	45(32.37)	27(40.3)	18(25.0)	0.31
eGFR(ml/min/1.73 m^2)	80.22±17.53	74.96±16.00	83.55±17.75	0.01

Table 1 (Continued)

Baseline characteristics	Total (n=139)	ALLO + (n = 67)	ALLO- (n = 72)	p (ALLO+/ ALLO-)
Peripheral - n(%)	18(12.9)	10(14.9)	8(11.1)	0.21
Carotid - n(%)	75(53.9)	40(59.7)	35(48.6)	0.08
LVH ECG/echo- n(%)	118(84.9)	55(82.1)	63(87.5)	0.13
Clinical organ damage-				
n(%)	23(16.6)	14(20.9)	9(12.5)	0.19
Renal	5(3.6)	3(4.5)	2(2.8)	0.63
Peripheral	11(7.9)	8(11.9)	3(4.2)	0.071
Cerebrovascular				
Coronary	57(41.0)	31(46.3)	26(36.1)	0.18
HF	12(8.6)	5(7.5)	7(9.7)	0.45
AF	14(10.1)	8(11.9)	6(8.3)	0.84
Hypertensive retinopathy ≥ gradeIII	23(16.6)	15(22.4)	8(11.1)	0.06
DM II- n(%)	27(19.4)	14 (20.9)	13 (18.1)	0.58
HT risk category - n(%)				0.21
Low	5(3.6)	2(2.9)	3(4.2)	
Moderate	29(20.9)	12(17.9)	17(23.6)	
High	56(40.3)	26(38.8)	30(41.7)	
Very high	49(35.3)	27(40.3)	22(30.6)	
Medication - n(%)				
ASA	66(47.5)	29(43.3)	37(51.4)	0.34
ACO	14(10.1)	8(11.9)	6(8.3)	0.48
Statin	80(57.6)	37(55.2)	43(59.7)	0.59
ACEI	88(63.3)	38(56.7)	50(69.4)	0.15
ARB	24(17.3)	11(16.4)	13(18.1)	0.80
Beta blockers	96(69.1)	45(67.2)	51(70.8)	0.64
Calcium channel blockers DHP	38(27.3)	17(25.4)	21(29.2)	0.62
Diuretics	69(49.6)	38(56.7)	31(41.1)	0.13
Central acting agents	8(5.8)	3(4.5)	5(6.9)	0.54
Antiarrhythmics (Amiodarone)	22(15.8)	14(20.9)	8(11.1)	0.12

F=female, M=male, n=number; SBP= systolic blood pressure; DBP=diastolic blood pressure; ABPM=ambulatory blood pressure monitoring; BMI=body mass index; DM II=type II diabetes mellitus; eGFR= estimated glomerular filtration rate; LVH = left ventricular hypertrophy; HF=heart failure; AF=atrial fibrillation; ASA=acetylsalicylic acid; ACO=oral anticoagulants; ACEI=angiotensin-converting-enzyme inhibitors; ARB=angiotensin receptors blockers; DHP=dihydropyridine.

Serum uric acid level (mg/dL) at the initial evaluation was similar in both groups of patients, with an average within normal limits: 5.43±2.22 in ALLO+ and 5.05±1.81 in ALLO- (p=0.26) and was significantly correlated to: the age of patients (r=0.49, p<0.0001), HT grade (r=0.32, p=0.0005), mean BP on ABPM, both systolic (r=0.31, p=0.041) and diastolic (r=0.39, p=0.0099), cardiovascular risk factors: waist circumference (r=0.39, p<0.0001) and the number of cardiovascular risk factors (r-0.35, p=0. 0001), target organ damage indices: glomerular filtration rate (r=-0.40, p<0.0001 – inverse correlation), carotid intima-media thickness (r=0.32, p=0.0006), left ventricular mass (r=0.37, p=0.0001) and left ventricular mass index (r=0.32, p=0.001).

The Effect of Allopurinol on Serum Uric Acid

In ALLO+ sUA (mg/dL) decreased significantly after one month, reaching 3.69±1.72 (p<0.0001), an average decrease of 30% from baseline and remained constant low at 3 months (3.74±1.06, p=0.73) and at 6 months (3.97±1.23, p=0.37) –Figure 1.

In ALLO- sUA (mg/dL) did not change significantly during the follow-up, reaching after a month 5.11±1.65 (p=0.18), after 3 months 5.18±1.55 (p=0.11) and after 6 months 5.24±1.34 (p=0.82).

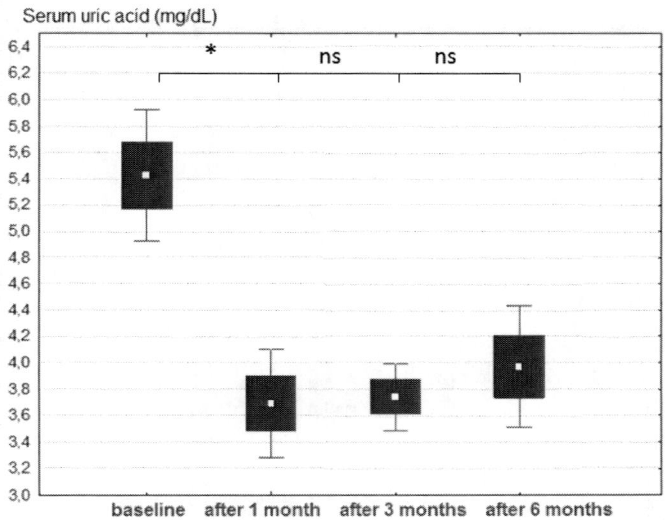

Figure 1. Serum uric acid variation in ALLO+.

The effect of allopurinol on blood pressure was automatically evaluated by ABPM, determining the mean systolic and diastolic BP/24 hours at baseline and after one month. In ALLO+ group BP values (mmHg) decreased significantly after a month: systolic BP (SBP) 138.96±14.95 to 135.23±13.03, a percentage reduction of 2.6% (p<0.0001) and diastolic BP (DBP) from 84.99±13.09 to 83.02±13.08, a percentage reduction of about 2% (p=0.003). In ALLO- group systolic BP (mmHg) decreased from 142.76±13.26 to 142.16±12.10, a percentage reduction of 0.34% (p=0.01), but far less than the decrease in ALLO + (p<0.0001) and diastolic BP (mmHg) changed insignificantly, from 88.25±14.57 to 87.95±13.79, by 0.2% (p=0.30).

The Effect of Allopurinol on Endothelial Function

At baseline endothelial function assessed as percent change in the diameter of the brachial artery (FMD (%)) was similar in both groups (10.56±6.54 in ALLO+ and 10.77±6.85 in ALLO-, p=0.71). In ALLO endothelial function was significantly improved after one month, FMD (%) increasing on average by 31%, to 13.43±6.41 (p<0.0001), remaining constant after 3 months (13.80±5.76, p=0.28), but with a significant improvement noted at 6 months (16.89±5.03, p=0.017) – Figure 2. In ALLO- endothelial function changed insignificantly, reaching after 1 month 10.74±6.41% (p=0.93), after 3 months 11.14±6.20% (p=0.30) and after 6 months 10.29±3.19% (p=0.3).

Endothelial function evaluated at baseline was inversely correlated with sUA in all patients (r=-0.35, p <0.0001) - Figure 3. Changes in endothelial function significantly correlated with changes in sUA in ALLO+: 0-1 month r=-0.30, p=0.026, 0-3 months r=-0.47, p<0.0001, 0-6 months r=-0.44, p=0.037.

Changes in endothelial function were analyzed according to the risk categories of HT [43] (2-moderate, 3-high, 4-very high). The effect of allopurinol on endothelial function was more important as the cardiovascular risk of patients was higher. Between 0-6 months, FMD (%) increased in ALLO+ in patients with HT with moderate risk by 3.52±4.05 (p=0.044), in patients with high risk by 3.20±3.51 (p=0.036), in patients with very high risk by 9.49±4.93 (p<0.0001) - Figure 4.

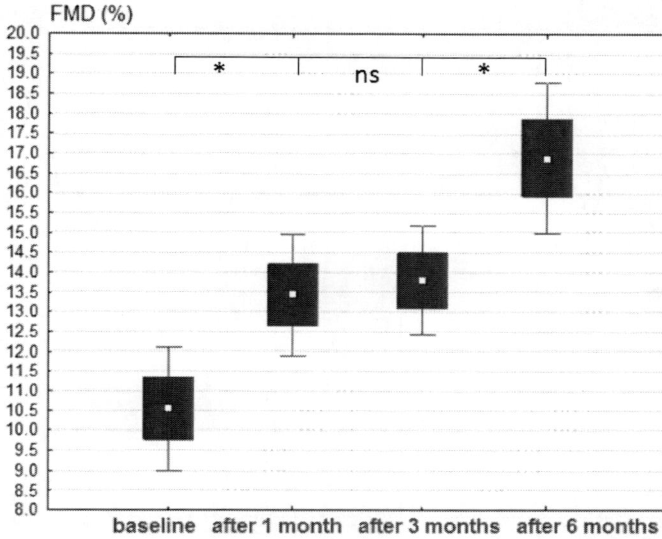

Figure 2. Variation of endothelial function in ALLO+.

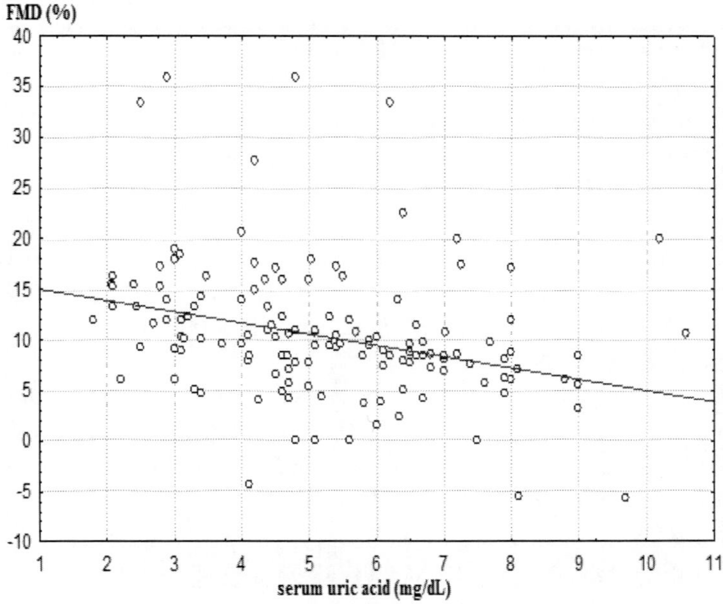

Figure 3. Correlation between FMD(%) and serum uric acid levels at baseline.

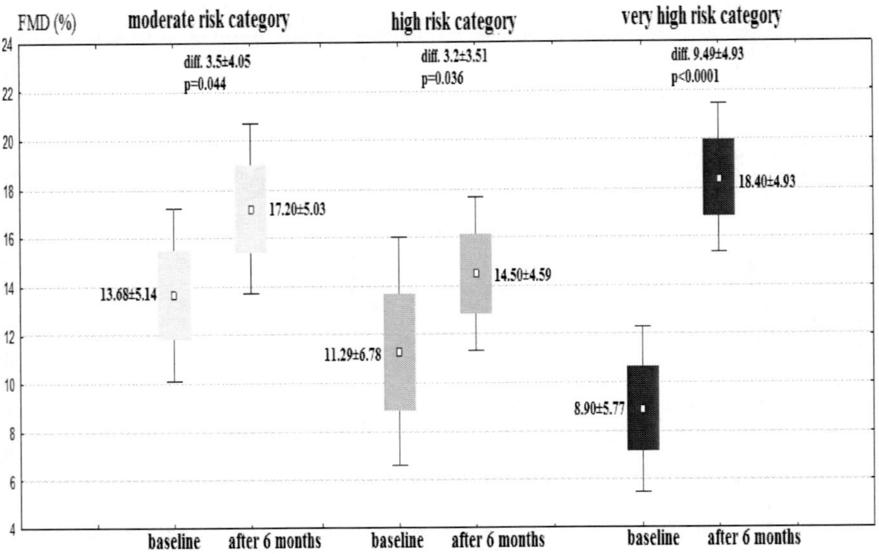

Figure 4. 0-6 months variation in endothelial function in ALLO+ according to HT risk category.

Effect of Allopurinol on Platelet Function

At baseline platelet function assessed by optical aggregometry method was similar in patients in the two groups. ADP aggregation (%) was 65.76±21.07 in ALLO+ and 63.12±27.14 in ALLO- (p=0.53). Collagen aggregation (%) was 75.61±23.13 in ALLO+ and 76.35±18.95 in ALLO- (p=0.84). After one month, ADP aggregation (%) decreased in ALLO+ by about 48%, to 34.64±23.56 (p<0.0001). In ALLO- ADP aggregation (%) increased by about 32%, to 70.26±21.09 (p<0.0001). After a month, aggregation to ADP was significantly lower in ALLO+ than in ALLO- (p<0.0001). After one month of treatment, collagen aggregation (%) significantly decreased in ALLO+, to 60.99±24.53, a decrease of about 18% (p<0.0001). In ALLO- collagen aggregation (%) did not change significantly, reaching 76.31±18.15 after one month (p=0.98). Collagen aggregation was significantly lower in ALLO+ than in ALLO- (p<0.0001) after one month.

The two groups were divided according to the concomitant acetylsalicylic acid (ASA) in treatment into four groups: ALLO+ASA+, ALLO+ASA-, ALLO-ASA+, ALLO-ASA-. Changes in platelet function were separately analyzed for each of the four groups (Table 2).

Table 2. Changes in platelet aggregation to ADP (%) and collagen (%) according to the presence of ASA in the regimen

	ALLO+ ASA+ (n=29)	p ALLO+ ASA+	ALLO- ASA+ (n=37)	p ALLO- ASA+	ALLO+ ASA- (n=38)	p ALLO+ ASA-	ALLO- ASA- (n=35)	p ALLO- ASA-
ADP Agg initial	57.41± 22.49		44.81± 22.38		71.03± 20.10		82.49± 16.03	
ADP Agg after 1 month	36.59± 17.31	**<0.0001**	56.94± 18.93	**0.05**	34.81± 28.06	**<0.0001**	84.34± 12.35	**0.19**
Collagen Agg initial	62.07± 24.92		67.32± 19.69		85.76± 15.35		85.89± 12.51	
Collagen Agg after 1 month	52.72± 23.82	**0.00031**	66.24± 18.29	**0.72**	67.11± 23.73	**<0.0001**	86.94± 10.34	**0.37**

Agg = maximum aggregation by optical aggregometry method (%); ADP = adenosine diphosphate

ADP Aggregation

At baseline patients treated with ASA had a lower level of platelet aggregation to ADP, both in ALLO+ (p=0.021), and in ALLO- (p<0.0001). After one month platelet aggregation to ADP decreased significantly in ALLO+, the decrease being significantly higher in patients who were not treated with ASA (p=0.046).

Collagen Aggregation

At baseline platelet aggregation to collagen was lower in patients who were treated with ASA, both in ALLO+ (p<0.0001), and in ALLO- (p<0.0001). After one month platelet aggregation to collagen decreased significantly in ALLO+, the decrease being similar irrespective of concomitant ASA treatment (p=0.08).

At baseline platelet aggregation to ADP and collagen were not correlated with sUA levels. In ALLO+ there were significant correlations between sUA variation and modification of platelet function in patients treated with ASA: for ADP aggregation r=0.44, p=0.034 and for collagen aggregation r=-0.57, p=0.0042.

DISCUSSION

The study group included patients with optimally treated HT, hyperuricemia was not among inclusion criteria. Most patients (74.1%) had normal sUA levels (mg/dl), which significantly decreased with allopurinol 300 mg/day. After one month of treatment, there was a maximum reduction in sUA levels, without additional decrease on continued allopurinol therapy, but sUA remained significantly lower compared to baseline. The data suggest that after reaching its maximal effect, allopurinol exerts a constant inhibition on uric acid synthesis. Serum uric acid levels varied slightly during the six month follow-up in the control group.

Long-term treatment with allopurinol has been reported to decrease uric acid levels by 32% after 12 months of follow-up in patients with hyperuricemia [54]. The different response of patients to the same dose of allopurinol and the influence of renal function on plasma levels of allopurinol could contribute to the inhomogeneity of the study data [55, 56]. However study results are similar with the results of larger cohort studies in which the confounding factors were excluded using multivariate analysis. The similar long-term medication in both study groups makes the possible influence of concomitant medication on sUA level unlikely.

In some patients in ALLO+ sUA has reached levels below 2 mg/dL, bringing into question the extent to which uricemia may fall and long-term impact of a low sUA level. In the treatment of gout the recommendation is to achieve a target sUA level ≤ 6mg/dL, aiming to keep its concentration below the molecule solubility in plasma and extracellular space (about 7 mg/dL) [57]. So far, there have been no clinical studies aimed to identify long-term consequences of sUA below 2 mg/dL, when hypouricemia diagnosis is considered, based on demographics. The only evidence came from a series of epidemiological studies, which suggested a possible protective effect of uric acid in neurodegenerative diseases, in particular multiple sclerosis and Parkinson disease [58, 59].

The effectiveness of allopurinol in lowering sUA in patients with hyperuricemia is similar to other hypouricemic drugs [54]. However, allopurinol has additional beneficial effects in patients with cardiovascular risk or established cardiovascular pathology.

Several studies had analyzed the effect of allopurinol on BP, with different results [32, 37, 60, 61, 62]. Agarwal et al. conducted a meta-analysis of 10 trials and concluded that allopurinol produces a slight but significant decrease in BP (SBP decreased by 3.3 mmHg and DBP by 1.3 mmHg) [63] In ALLO+

group SBP decreased after one month by 3.73±3.03 mmHg (p <0.0001) and DBP by 1.97 ± 4.60 mmHg (p = 0.003). Feig et al. demonstrated that allopurinol 400 mg/day decreased SBP by 6.3 mmHg and DBP by 4.6 mmHg after 2 weeks in a group of adolescents with hyperuricemia, newly onset HT and without antihypertensive therapy [32]. In animal models it had been demonstrated that the hyperuricemia can induce hypertension by inflammatory changes in the renal microcirculation, activation of the renin-angiotensin system and endothelial dysfunction [64, 65]. In this stage of disease, BP can be reduced by lowering sUA level. The persistence of elevated BP and consecutive ischemic renal vasoconstriction generates chronic intrinsic renal and systemic inflammation. Persistent hyperuricemia maintains renal impairment by inducing renal vasoconstriction secondary to renin-angiotensin system activation and proliferation of smooth muscle cells [2]. Kidney damage caused by the combined effect of HT and hyperuricemia contributes to the progression of HT and maintains the increased sUA level by decreased renal excretion [66]. In this advanced stage of the disease, lowering sUA would not be associated with significantly decrease in BP values [8]. This may explain the small effect of allopurinol on BP in patients with long term HT and hyperuricemia.

Although at baseline BP values correlated with sUA, there was no correlation between BP variation and sUA change. The lowering BP effect of allopurinol probably consisted of the inhibition of xanthine oxidase, a key enzyme for oxidative metabolism, which is one of the pathophysiological substrate of the HT progression. The effect of allopurinol on BP was observed in patients with optimal BP control, suggesting an ongoing relationship between HT and oxidative stress, lowered by allopurinol together with reduced uric acid synthesis. Since the two groups had similar profiles, it has been hypothesized that the BP differences observed after one month are due exclusively to allopurinol treatment.

The study results confirmed that allopurinol improved endothelial function in hypertensive patients with optimal therapeutic control, the more important as the severity of HT was higher. The improvement in endothelial function was progressive, suggesting a continuous effect of allopurinol. Literature does not provide evidence on long term effect of allopurinol treatment on endothelial function [67, 68]. A recent meta-analysis, included 11 trials, supporting the effect of allopurinol to improve endothelial function after a follow up period of maximum 4 months [15].

Endothelial function in the control group did not change significantly during follow-up, suggesting that long-term antihypertensive treatment is only able to improve endothelial function up to a limited extent. Compared to statins, angiotensin II converting enzyme inhibitors or spironolactone, high doses of allopurinol may have a more significant effect on endothelial function even in patients already treated with these drugs [37].

In the study group, mean baseline FMD was within normal limits and inversely correlated with sUA. Endothelial dysfunction is an important predictor for HT development, target organ damage and the occurrence of cardiovascular events [37, 69, 70]. The mechanisms of endothelial dysfunction are complex and there is important evidence supporting the involvement of uric acid in endothelial dysfunction [69, 71]. It has been experimentally shown that uric acid decreases the bioavailability of nitric oxide and mediates endothelial dysfunction in animal models [72, 73]. Reports in the literature confirm the inverse correlation between sUA levels and endothelial dysfunction, a consequence of uric acid involvement in oxidative metabolism [9, 67, 68]. Similarly to the literature data, sUA level in the study group was significantly correlated with cardiovascular risk factors and hypertensive target organ damage, confirming its association with cardiovascular risk [2, 3, 4, 5, 6, 7].

In patients treated with allopurinol the change in endothelial function was inversely correlated with changes in sUA level. Previous studies suggested that the effect of allopurinol on endothelial function improvement is due to the reduction of vascular oxidative stress, and not to the decrease in sUA *per se* [37]. Using equivalent doses of allopurinol (300 mg) and probenecid (1000 mg), it has been proved that probenecid had no effect on endothelial function at similar sUA decrease, supporting the allopurinol effect of lowering oxidative stress [37].

The effect of allopurinol on endothelial function was higher as HT severity (assessed by the cardiovascular risk category) increased. It has been suggested that HT is not the essential factor involved in endothelial dysfunction. In a group of patients with diabetes and mild HT, after multivariate statistical analysis, the effect of allopurinol on endothelial function was influenced by the presence of diabetes, hypercholesterolemia and lastly by HT [19].

Oxidative stress and inflammation activation contribute directly or through endothelial dysfunction to the prothrombotic status associated with HT, with important consequences on target organ damage, prognosis and treatment [35]. By decreasing free radicals generation, allopurinol reduces oxidative stress, but there are no data related to its effects on platelet function. In an experimental study performed in a canine model (n = 10) the antiplatelet effect of allopurinol was demonstrated in vitro, by decreasing platelet aggregation to ADP measured by the optical aggregometry from 48.3 ± 1.3 to 24.8 ± 1.5%, p <0.0001 [74].

In the present study, the treatment with allopurinol 300 mg/day for one month significantly decreased platelet aggregation to ADP and collagen in patients with HT with optimal therapeutic control. The allopurinol antiplatelet effect was partly independent of the sUA-lowering effect.

Patients who were initially treated with ASA had a lower level of platelet aggregation to ADP and collagen, indicating normal response to antiplatelet therapy.

There was a significant decrease in the maximum percentage of aggregation to ADP in all patients treated with allopurinol 300 mg/day, comparable to the antiaggregant response to clopidogrel [75, 76, 77]. The majority of patients in ALLO+ group could be considered "responders," reaching a rate of ADP aggregation below 30% after a month of treatment with allopurinol.

A significant decrease in the percentage of aggregation to collagen was noted in patients treated with allopurinol, but this effect was comparable to the ASA response only a small number of patients [78].

Concomitant treatment with ASA influenced the effect of allopurinol on platelet aggregation, patients without concomitant treatment with ASA having a higher decrease in aggregation to ADP and collagen. It has been shown that there is a decreased platelet sensitivity in chronic treatment with ASA, suggesting alternative pathways of thromboxane A2 (TXA 2) or other platelet agonists synthesis [78].

Platelet function assessed by the maximum percentage of aggregation did not correlate with sUA levels at baseline. The literature data are controversial, several studies proving that hyperuricemia does not affect platelet function and does not induce a prothrombotic status, while the results of an experimental study have shown an increased in platelets aggregation associated with induced hyperuricemia [39, 80, 81]. It was demonstrated that hyperuricemia is associated with decreased ADP degradation, which stimulates platelet aggregation, but, proving that platelets phagocytize urate molecules, it was presumed that uric acid may have also a direct effect on platelets [38]. More recent studies have shown that uric acid may increase the metabolism of arachidonic acid in platelets and the pro-inflammatory status associated with hyperuricemia may contribute to platelet activation [81, 82]. In the present study, the lack of correlation between changes in platelet aggregation and sUA may be related to normal sUA level in most patients, while increased platelets aggregation has been shown in hyperuricemia, suggesting a direct effect of allopurinol on platelets. This hypothesis should be demonstrated in further studies including a higher number of patients with extended follow-up period. The mechanism of allopurinol effect on platelets aggregation should be considered in the framework of the complex link between uric acid and oxidative stress, which may cause progression of atherosclerotic lesions and thrombotic events.

CONCLUSION

In patients with hypertension optimally treated, allopurinol therapy persistently decreased serum uric acid and slightly but significantly lowered blood pressure. The endothelial function was significantly improved by allopurinol treatment, particularly in patients with higher cardiovascular risk. The antiplatelet effect of allopurinol was proven by decreasing platelet aggregation both to ADP and collagen.

Given the complexity of the relationship between high blood pressure, oxidative stress and uric acid, complementary treatment with allopurinol could prevent the progression to organ damage and cardiovascular events in HT patients. However, new evidence is needed to support the allopurinol treatment in HT patients with normal serum uric acid levels.

REFERENCES

[1] Mohamed FA. On chronic Bright's disease, and its essential symptoms. *Lancet* 1879;1:399–401.

[2] Feig DI, Kang DH, Johnson RJ. Uric acid and cardiovascular risk. *N Engl J Med.* 2008;359:1811–1821.

[3] Fang J, Alderman MH. Serum uric acid and cardiovascular mortality: the NHANES I epidemiologic follow-up study, 1971-1992. *JAMA.* 2000;283:2404-2410.

[4] Niskanen LK, Laaksonen DE, Nyyssonen K, et al. Uric acid level as a risk factor for cardiovascular and all-cause mortality in middle-aged men: a prospective cohort study. *Arch Intern Med* 2004;164:1546-51.

[5] Liese AD, Hense HW, Lowel H, Doring A, Tietze M, Keil U. Association of serum uric acid with all-cause and cardiovascular disease mortality and incident myocardial infarction in the MONICA Augsburg cohort: World Health Organization Monitoring Trends and Determinants in Cardiovascular Diseases. *Epidemiology* 1999;10:391–7.

[6] Verdecchia P, Schillaci G, Reboldi G, Santeusanio F, Porcellati C, Brunetti P. Relation between serum uric acid and risk of cardiovascular disease in essential hypertension: the PIUMA study. *Hypertension* 2000;36:1072–8.

[7] Nakagawa T, Tuttle KR, Short RA, Johnson RJ. Hypothesis:fructose-induced hyperuricemia as a casual mechanism for the epidemic of the metabolic syndrome. *Nat Clin Pract Nephrol* 2005; 1: 80-86.

[8] Mazzali M, Hughes J, Kim YG, et al. Elevated uric acid increases blood pressure in the rat by a novel crystal-independent mechanism. *Hypertension.* 2001;38(5):1101-1106.

[9] Sanchez-Lozada LG, Rivard C, Lanaspa M, Roncal C, Franco M, Sautin Y, et al: Uric acid alters mitochondrial biogenesis in cultured human endothelial cells. *Am Soc Nephrol Annual Meeting,* 2009, abstract.

[10] Ilieşiu A, Dusceac D, Câmpeanu A. Serum uric acid in cardiovascular disease. *MAEDICA Journal of Cilnical Medicine* 2010; 5(8): 186-192.

[11] Câmpeanu A, Olinescu R, Nistorescu Diana, Zaharia O. Relationship between oxidative stress and C-reactive protein and myocardial dysfunction in chronic heart failure of ischemic etiology. *Eur J Heart Fail* 2002; 1: 1-11

[12] Dzau V, Braunwald E. Resolved and unresolved issues in the prevention and treatment of coronary artery disease: a workshop consensus statement. *Am Heart J.* 1991;121:1244–1263.

[13] Lippi G, Montagnana M, Franchini M, Favaloro EJ, Targher G. The paradoxical relationship between serum uric acid and cardiovascular disease. *Clinica Chimica Acta* 392 (2008) 1–7.

[14] Whiteman M, Ketsawatsakul U, Halliwell B. A reassessment of the peroxynitrite scavenging activity of uric acid. *Ann NY Acad Sci* 2002;962:242–259.

[15] Kanbay M, Siriopol D, Nistor I, Elcioglu OC, Telci O, Takir M, Johnson RJ, Covic A. Effects of allopurinol on endothelial dysfunction: a meta-analysis. *Am J Nephrol* 2014;39:348–356.

[16] Guthikonda S, Sinkey C, Barenz T, Haynes WG. Xanthine oxidase inhibition reverses endothelial dysfunction in heavy smokers. *Circulation.* 2003;107:416–421.

[17] Yiginer O, Ozcelik F, Inanc T, Aparci M, Ozmen N, Cingozbay BY, et al: Allopurinol improves endothelial function and reduces oxidant-inflammatory enzyme of myeloperoxidase in metabolic syndrome. *Clin Res Cardiol* 2008; 97: 334–340.

[18] Dogan A, Yarlioglues M, Kaya MG, Karadag Z, Dogan S, Ardic I, et al: Effect of long-term and high-dose allopurinol therapy on endothelial function in normotensive diabetic patients. *Blood Press* 2011; 20: 182–187.

[19] Butler R, Morris AD, Belch JJ, Hill A, Struthers AD: Allopurinol normalizes endothelial dysfunction in type 2 diabetics with mild hypertension. *Hypertension* 2000; 35: 746–751.

[20] El Solh AA, Saliba R, Bosinski T, Grant BJ, Berbary E, Miller N: Allopurinol improves endothelial function in sleep apnoea: a randomised controlled study. *Eur Respir J* 2006;27: 997–1002.

[21] Yelken B, Caliskan Y, Gorgulu N, Altun I,Yilmaz A, Yazici H, et al: Reduction of uric acid levels with allopurinol treatment improves endothelial function in patients with chronic kidney disease. *Clin Nephrol* 2012; 77:275–282.

[22] Goicoechea M, de Vinuesa SG, Verdalles U, Ruiz-Caro C, Ampuero J, Rincon A, et al: Effect of allopurinol in chronic kidney disease progression and cardiovascular risk. *Clin J Am Soc Nephrol* 2010; 5: 1388–1393.

[23] Noman A, Ang DS, Ogston S, et al. Effect of high-dose allopurinol on exercise in patients with chronic stable angina: a randomised, placebo controlled crossover trial. *Lancet.* 2010;375:2161–2167.

[24] Rajendra NS, Ireland S, George J, Belch JJ, Lang CC, Struthers AD: Mechanistic insights into the therapeutic use of high-dose allopurinol in angina pectoris. *J Am Coll Cardiol* 2011; 58: 820–828.

[25] Farquharson CA, Butler R, Hill A, Belch JJ, Struthers AD: Allopurinol improves endothelial dysfunction in chronic heart failure. *Circulation* 2002; 106: 221–226.

[26] Doehner W, Schoene N, Rauchhaus M, Leyva-Leon F, Pavitt DV, Reaveley DA, et al: Effectsof xanthine oxidase inhibition with allopurinol on endothelial function and peripheral blood flow in hyperuricemic patients with chronic heart failure: results from two placebo-controlled studies. *Circulation* 2002;105: 2619–2624.

[27] Dusceac D, Iliesiu A, Campeanu Al. Effects of high dose Allopurinol on endothelial dysfunction, serum uric acid, oxidative stress, and inflammation in chronic heart failure. [Efectele allopurinolului în doze mari asupra disfuncţiei endoteliale, acidului uric seric, stresului oxidativ şi inflamaţiei în insuficienţa cardiacă cronică.] *Medicina Moderna* 2013; 20: 7.

[28] Câmpeanu A, Ilieşiu A, Nistorescu D, Străjean B, Uscoiu G, Dusceac D, Nanea IT. Serum uric acid levels in patients with recent decompensated heart failure - a new biomarker?. *Eur J Heart Fail Supplements* (2010) 9, S35.

[29] Câmpeanu A, Ilieşiu Adriana, Moldoveanu Elena, Dusceac D, Uscoiu Gabriela, Marta Delia. The relationship between uric acid, oxidativ stress and inflammation in chronic heart failure. *Eur J Heart Fail Supplements.* 2011, 10, suppl 1, S150-151.

[30] Câmpeanu A, Ilieşiu A, Dusceac D, Moldoveanu E. Effects of high dose Allopurinol on serum uric acid, biomarkers of oxidative stress, inflammation and cardiac remodeling in chronic heart failure. [Efectele allopurinolului în doze mari asupra acidului uric seric şi a biomarkerilor de stress oxidativ, inflamaţie şi remodelare miocardică, în insuficienţa cardiacă cronică] - *Rom J Cardiology,* 2012,Supliment 183.

[31] Câmpeanu A, Ilieşiu A, Uscoiu G, Dusceac D, Cristea A, Marta D, Moldoveanu E. Effects of high dose allopurinol on serum uric acid, oxidative stress and inflammatory biomarkers in patients with chronic heart failure. *Eu J Heart Failure* 2013 (15)S1, S148.

[32] Feig DI, Soletsky B, Johnson RJ: Effect of allopurinol on blood pressure of adolescents with newly diagnosed essential hypertension: a randomized trial. *JAMA* 2008; 300: 924–932.

[33] Soletsky B, Feig DI: Uric acid reduction rectifies prehypertension in obese adolescents. *Hypertension* 2012; 60: 1148–1156.

[34] Kanbay M, Solak Y, Gaipov A, Takir M, Weiner DE. Allopurinol as a Kidney-Protective, Cardioprotective, and Antihypertensive Agent: Hype or Reality? *Blood Purif* 2014;37:172–178.

[35] Lip GY. Hypertension, Platelets, and the Endothelium: The “Thrombotic Paradox” of Hypertension (or “Birmingham Paradox”) Revisited. *Hypertensio*n 2003; 41: 199-200.

[36] Davi G, Patrono C. Platelet Activation and Atherothrombosis. *N Engl J Med* 2007;357:2482-94.

[37] George J, Carr E, Davies J, et al. High-dose allopurinol improves endothelial function by profoundly reducing vascular oxidative stress and not by lowering uric acid. *Circulation.* 2006;114:2508–251.

[38] Wildeman, Richard Albert, "Effects Of Allopurinol On Platelet Function In Man And Experimental Animals" (1976). *Digitized Theses.* Paper 915.

[39] Ciompi ML, DeCaterina R, Bertolucci D, Bernini W, Michelassi C: Uric acid levels and platelet function in humans. An in-vivo ex-vivo study. *Clin Exp Rheumatol* 1983 Apr-Jun;1(2):143-7.

[40] Hodorogea AS, Câmpeanu A, Uscătescu V, Nanea IT. Effects of Allopurinol on platelet function in essential arterial hypertension – a preliminary study. [Efectele allopurinolului asupra funcției plachetare în hipertensiunea arterială esențială - studiu preliminary]. *Medicina Internă* 2014 (XI) 5: 25-36.

[41] Câmpeanu A, Hodorogea AS, Uscătescu V, Nanea IT: Effect of allopurinol on serum uric acid and platelet aggregation in patients with essential arterial hypertension. *European Heart Journal* 2015 36: 1102-1102.

[42] Macfarlane DG, Slade R, Hopes PA, Hartog MH: A study of platelet aggregation and adhesion in gout. *Clin Exp Rheumatol.* 1983 Jan-Mar;1(1):63-6.

[43] The Task Force for the management of arterial hypertension of the European Society of Hypertension (ESH) and of the European Society of Cardiology (ESC). 2013 ESH/ESC Guidelines for the management of arterial hypertension. *European Heart Journal* 2013: 34;2159–2219.

[44] Charakida M,Masi S, Thomas F. Luscher Th. F, Kastelein JP, Deanfield JE: Assessment of atherosclerosis: the role of flow-mediated dilatation: *European Heart Journal* 2010. 31: 2854–2861.

[45] Thijssen DH, Black MA, Pyke KE, Padilla J, Atkinson G, Harris RA, Parker B, Widlansky ME, Tschakovsky ME, Green DJ. Assessment of flowmediated dilation in humans: a methodological and physiological guideline. *Am J Physiol Heart Circ Physiol* 300: H2–H12, 2011.

[46] Harris RA, Nishiyama SK, Wray DW, Richardson RS. Ultrasound assessment of flow-mediated dilation. *Hypertension.* 2010;55:1075-1085.

[47] Donald AE, Halcox JP, Charakida M, et al. Methodological approaches to optimize reproducibility and power in clinical studies of flow-mediated dilation. *J Am Coll Cardiol* 2008;51: 1959–1964.

[48] Vogel RA - Coronary Risk Factors, Endothelial Function, and Atherosclerosis: *A Review Clin. Cardiol.* 1997; 2: 426-432.

[49] Zhou L, Schmaier AH. Platelet Aggregation Testing in Platelet-Rich Plasma. Description of Procedures With the Aim to Develop Standards in the Field. *Am J Clin Pathol* 2005;123:172-183.

[50] Catherine Hayward, Karen A. Moffat, Anne Raby, Sara Israels, Elizabeth Plumhoff, Flynn Zehnder JL. Development of North American Consensus Guidelines for Medical Laboratories That Perform and Interpret Platelet Function Testing Using Light Transmission Aggregometry. *Am J Clin Pathol* 2010;134:955-963.

[51] Cattaneo M, Cerletti C, Harrison P, Hayward CPM, Kenny D, Nugent D, Nurden P, Rao AK, Schmaier AH, Watson SP, Lussana F, Pugliano MT, Michelson AD. Recommendations for the Standardization of Light Transmission Aggregometry: A Consensus of the Working Party from the Platelet Physiology Subcommittee of SSC/ISTH. *J Thromb Haemost* 2013; 11:1183-1189.

[52] Linnemann B, Schwonberg J, Mani H, Prochnow S, Lindhoff-Last E. Standardization of light transmittance aggregometry for monitoring antiplatelet therapy: an adjustment for platelet count is not necessary. *J Thromb Haemost* 2008; 6: 677 – 683.

[53] Mani H, Luxembourg B, Klaffling C, Erbe M, Lindhoff-Last E. Use of native or platelet count adjusted platelet rich plasma for platelet aggregation measurements. *J Clin Pathol* 2005; 58:747 – 750.

[54] Becker MA, Schumacher HR, MacDonald PA, Lloyd E, Lademacher C. Clinical efficacy and safety of successful longterm urate lowering with febuxostat or allopurinol in subjects with gout. *J Rheumatol.* 2009 Jun; 36(6):1273–82.

[55] Hoskison TK, Wortmann RL. Advances in the management of gout and hyperuricaemia. *Scand J Rheumatol.* 2006;35(4):251–60.

[56] Dalbeth N, Stamp L. Allopurinol dosing in renal impairment: walking the tightrope between adequate urate lowering and adverse events. *Semin Dial.* 2007;20(5):391–5.

[57] Zhang W, Doherty M, Bardin T, Pascual E, Barskova V, Conaghan P, Gerster J, Jacobs J, Leeb B, Liote F, et al. EULAR evidence based recommendations for gout. Part II: Management. Report of a task force of the EULAR Standing Committee for International Clinical Studies Including Therapeutics (ESCISIT). *Ann Rheum Dis* 2006;65:1312–1324.

[58] Weisskopf MG, O'Reilly E, Chen H, Schwarzschild MA, Ascherio A. Plasma urate and risk of Parkinson's disease. *Am J Epidemiol* 2007;166:561–567.
[59] Rentzos M, Nikolaou C, Anagnostouli M, Rombos A, Tsakanikas K, Economou M, Dimitrakopoulos A, Karouli M, Vassilopoulos D. Serum uric acid and multiple sclerosis. *Clin Neurol Neurosurg* 2006;108:527–531.
[60] Kanbay M, Ozkara A, Selcoki Y, et al. Effect of treatment of hyperuricemia with allopurinol on blood pressure, creatinine clearence, and proteinuria in patients with normal renal functions. *Int Urol Nephrol.* 2007;39:1227–1233.
[61] Kanbay M, Huddam B, Azak A, et al. A randomized study of allopurinol on endothelial function and estimated glomular filtration rate in asymptomatic hyperuricemic subjects with normal renal function. *Clin J Am Soc Nephrol.* 2011;6:1887–1894.
[62] Khan F, George J, Wong K, et al. Allopurinol treatment reduces arterial wave reflection in stroke survivors. *Cardiovasc Ther.* 2008;26:247–252.
[63] Agarwal V, Hans N, Messerli FH. Effect of Allopurinol on Blood Pressure: A Systematic Review and Meta-Analysis *J Clin Hypertens* (Greenwich). 2013;15:435–442.
[64] Johnson RJ, Kang DH, Feig O, et al. Is there a pathogenetic role for uric acid in hypertension and cardiovascular and renal disease? *Hypertension* 2003;41:1183–90.
[65] Mazzali M, M, SegalMS, et al.Uric acidand hypertension: cause or effect? *Curr Rheumatol Rep* 2010;12:108–17.
[66] Johnson RJ, Herrera-Acosta J, Schreiner GF, Rodriguez-Iturbe B. Subtle acquired renal injury as a mechanism of salt-sensitive hypertension. *N. Engl. J. Med.* 2002; 346:913-923.
[67] Hodorogea AS, Câmpeanu A, Nanea IT, Gheorghe GS, Nicolae C, Ciobanu A. Relationship between serum uric acid, endothelial dysfunction and arterial hypertension severity – the role of allopurinol. [Relațiile dintre acidul uric seric, disfuncția endotelială și severitatea hipertensiunii arteriale - rolul alopurinolului]. *Medicina Internă* 2015 (XII) 2:21-35.
[68] Hodorogea AS, Câmpeanu A, Ilieşiu AM, Nanea IT. Effect of allopurinol on serum uric acid and endothelial function in patients with essential arterial hypertension optimally treated. *European Heart Journal* 2015; 36: 880-880.

[69] Mercuro G, Vitale C, Cerquetani E, Zoncu S, Deidda M, Fini M, et al: Effect of hyperuricemia upon endothelial function in patients at increased cardiovascular risk. *Am J Cardiol* 2004; 94: 932–935.

[70] Yiginer O, Ozcelik F, Inanc T, Aparci M, Ozmen N, Cingozbay BY, et al: Allopurinol improves endothelial function and reduces oxidant-inflammatory enzyme of myeloperoxidase in metabolic syndrome. *Clin Res Cardiol* 2008; 97: 334–340.

[71] Zoccali C, Maio R, Mallamaci F, Sesti G, Perticone F: Uric acid and endothelial dysfunction in essential hypertension. *J Am Soc Nephrol* 2006; 17: 1466–1471.

[72] Khosla UM, Zharikov S, Finch JL, Nakagawa T, Roncal C, Mu W, et al: Hyperuricemia induces endothelial dysfunction. *Kidney Int* 2005; 67: 1739–1742.

[73] Gersch C, Palii SP, Kim KM, Angerhofer A, Johnson RJ, Henderson GN: Inactivation of nitric oxide by uric acid. *Nucleosides Nucleotides Nucleic Acids* 2008; 27: 967–978.

[74] Kuwano K, Ikeda H, Oda T, et al: Xanthine oxidase mediates cyclic flow variations in a canine model of coronary arterial thrombosis. AJP - Heart June 1, 1996 vol. 270 no. 6 H1993-H1999.

[75] Gurbel PA, Becker RC, Mann KG, Steinhubl SR, Michelson AD. Platelet function monitoring in patients with coronary artery disease. *J Am Coll Cardiol* 2007;50:1822–34.

[76] 132. Gurbel PA, Bliden KP, Hiatt BL, O'Connor CM. Clopidogrel for coronary stenting: response variability, drug resistance, and the effect of pretreatment platelet reactivity. *Circulation* 2003;107:2908 –13.

[77] Gurbel PA, Antonino MJ, Bliden KP, et al. Platelet reactivity to adenosine diphosphate and long-term ischemic event occurrence following percutaneous coronary intervention: a potential antiplatelet therapeutic target. *Platelets* 2008;19:595– 604.

[78] Helgason CM et al. Aspirin response and failure in cerebral infarction. *Stroke.* 1993;24:345-350.

[79] Pulcinelli FM et al. Inhibition of Platelet Aggregation by Aspirin Progressively Decreases in Long-Term Treated Patients. *J Am Coll Cardiol* 2004;43: 979–84.

[80] Macfarlane DG, Slade R, Hopes PA, Hartog MH: A study of platelet aggregation and adhesion in gout. *Clin Exp Rheumatol.* 1983 Jan-Mar;1(1):63-6.

[81] Magda H M Youssef Is Hyperuricemia a Risk Factor to Cardiovascular Disease? http://dx.doi.org/10.5772/548714.

[82] Serhan, G. C, Lunberg, U, Weissmann, G. and Samuelsson, B. Formation of leukotriens and hydroxyl acids by human neutrophils and platelets exposed to monosodium urate. *Prostaglandins* 1984; 4:563.

BIOGRAPHICAL SKETCH

Andreea Simona Hodorogea

Affiliation:

"Carol Davila" University of Medicine and Pharmacy, "Theodor Burghele" Clinical Hospital, Department of Internal Medicine and Cardiology, Bucharest, Romania

Education:

2010- 2015,"Carol Davila" University of Medicine and Pharmacy, Bucharest: PhD in Medicine - European scholarship financed from the European Social Found and by the Romanian Government, thesis title *"Efects of Allopurinol on endothelial, hemodynamic and platelet function in patients with essential arterial hypertension"*

2005-2011, Romanian Ministry of Health, Residency Training Program: Cardiology Specialist

1998-2004,"Carol Davila" University of Medicine and Pharmacy, Bucharest: Medical Doctor, Confirmed as Cardiology Resident by National Residency Competition – december 2004

1994-1998, "Ion Creangă" National College, Bucharest: certified professional computer programmer, analyst and operator

Research and Professional Experience:

October 2011 – present: Teaching Assistant - Internal Medicine Discipline, Cardiology Specialist "Carol Davila" University of Medicine and Pharmacy, Bucharest, Faculty of Medicine;"Prof. Dr. Th. Burghele" Clinical Hospital Internal Medicine and Cardiology Department

2005 -2011 – Cardiology Resident: Clinical Cardiology, Cardiovascular angiography and catheterization, Cardiovascular surgery Echocardiography, Epidemiology, Research, Preveventive Cardiology, Anaestesia and Intensive Care, Internal Medicine Internships

Professional Appointments:

- Secretary of the Romanian Society of Cardiology -Bucharest branch
- Member of the Romanian Society of Cardiology and the European Society of Cardiology
- Collaboration within the editorial staff of the journal "Foaie de Informare Medicală"
- Co investigator RELAX 2 -A multicenter, randomized, double-blind, placebo-controlled phase IIIb study to evaluate the efficacy, safety and tolerability of Serelaxin when added to standard therapy in acute heart failure patients
- Co investigator RESTORE SR - LGN-VN-003: A multi-center, Randomized, double-blind, placebo-controlled study to Evaluate the Safety and efficacy of a single oral dose of vanoxerine for The conversion Of subjects with REcent onset atrial fibrillation or flutter to normal Sinus Rhythm
- Participation in the research team of the project IMUNOPLAT (Micro Immunosensors Platform for Metabolic Syndrome Investigation), winner within the Program PARTENERIATE – Collaborative Applied Research Projects– 2011 competition, funded by the Romanian Ministry of Education, Research, Youth and Sports by the Executive Unit for Higher Education Research Development and Innovation funding (UEFISCIDI)

Co-author of book chapters

1. Laura Bianca Drăghici, Andreea Simona Hodorogea, Cristina Bratiloveanu, Irina Andrei, S. Băilă, I.T. Nanea. " The left common carotid artery occlusion - asymptomatic" - Imaging in cardiac patients: page book to computer screen / edited by Carmen Ginghină, Bucharest: Editura Medicală 2015, ISBN: 978-973-39-0749-7
2. Ana Ciobanu, Maria Deaconu, Anca Popa, Andreea Simona Hodorogea, Gabriela Gheorghe, Denisa Predețeanu, Ioana Smărăndița Lacău, Camelia Nicolae, I.T. Nanea: "Dyspnoea of multiple etiology in multiple sclerosis" - Imaging in cardiac patients: page book to computer screen / edited by Carmen Ginghină, Bucharest: Editura Medicală 2014, ISBN: 978-973-39-0749-7
3. Ana Cristea, Delia Drăghici, Andreea Liteanu, Andreea Simona Hodorogea, Gabriela Gheorghe, Natalia Pătrașcu, A. Deutsch, R. Vătășescu, I.T. Nanea: " Cerebral embolism in a patient with dilated

cardiomyopathy, sinus rhythm resynchronization therapy and optimal anticoagulation" - Imaging in cardiac patients: page book to computer screen / edited by Carmen Ginghină, Bucharest: Editura Medicală 2013, ISBN: 978-973-39-0749-7

Papers published in extenso

1. Nanea IT, Nicolae C, Hodorogea AS, Slovenski M, Gheorghe GS. Systolic anterior motion and crossover of both mitral leaflets in hypertrophic cardiomyopathy Revista Română de Cardiologie 2016 (26) 1:3 2-33
2. Nicolae C, Pîrvu I, Hodorogea AS, Nanea IT, Ilieşiu AM, Gheorghe GS. Comorbidities of elderly patients with non-valvular atrial fibrillation and permanent anticoagulation with vitamin K antagonists decision in medical practice. Medicina Internă 2015 (XII) 6
3. Hodorogea AS, Câmpeanu A, Nanea IT, Gabriela Silvia Gheorghe, Camelia Nicolae, Ana Ciobanu. Relations between serum uric acid, endothelial dysfunction and severity of hypertension - the role of allopurinol. Medicina Internă 2015 (XII) 2:21-35
4. Hodorogea AS, Câmpeanu A, Uscătescu V, Nanea IT. Allopurinol effects on platelet function in essential hypertension - preliminary study. Medicina Internă 2014 (XI) 5: 25-36
5. Ciobanu A, Hodorogea AS, Ababei M, Gheorghe GS, Nanea IT. Variability of sinus rhythm in relation to the type of left ventricular hypertrophy and blood pressure profile in arterial hypertension. Medicina Internă 2014 (XI)1: 29-37
6. Ciobanu A, Hodorogea AS, Ababei M, Gheorghe GS, Ilieşiu AM, Uscoiu G, Nicolae C, Nanea IT. Dispersion of ventricular repolarization in relation to blood pressure values in essential hypertension. Medicina Modernă 2014 (21) 3:150-157
7. Gheorghe GS, Hodorogea AS, Nanea IT. "Statins - from bench to bedside." Revista Română de Cardiologie 2014 (24):3, 170-178
8. Mirescu MR, Nicolae C, Gheorghe G, Ciobanu A, Hodorogea AS, Almarichi S, Onceanu S, Ginghină C, Țintoiu I, Nanea IT. "The evolution of electrocardiographic changes in ST segment elevation myocardial infarction during the optimal therapeutic decision interval." Revista Română de Cardiologie 2014 (24):3, 163-170

Abstracts presented at international conferences published in ISI papers

1. GS Gheorghe, IT Nanea, AS Hodorogea, AM Ilieşiu. Prognostic value of Minnesota index determined at discharge after acute decompensated congestive heart failure. European Journal of Heart Failure 2016; 18: 195-195
2. Hodorogea AS, Câmpeanu A, Ilieşiu AM, Nanea IT. Effect of allopurinol on serum uric acid and endothelial function in patients with essential arterial hypertension optimally treated. European Heart Journal 2015; 36: 880-880
3. Câmpeanu A, Hodorogea AS, Uscătescu V, Nanea IT: Effect of allopurinol on serum uric acid and platelet aggregation in patients with essential arterial hypertension. European Heart Journal 2015 36: 1102-1102
4. Gheorghe GS, Nanea IT, Hodorogea AS, Ilieşiu AM. INR variability in the elderly with nonvalvular atrial fibrilaltion and decompensated heart failure. European Journal of Heart Failure 2015; 17: 304-304
5. Gheorghe GS, Hodorogea AS, Nanea IT, Gheorghe ACD: Comorbidities in the elderly with atrial fibrillation and the decision of oral anticoagulation in the real world – European Journal of Internal Medicine 2013 (24), S1, e9
6. Gheorghe GS, Cristea A, Liteanu A, Aramă D, Hodorogea AS, Nanea IT. T peak- T end interval and severe ventricular arrhythmia in patients with atrial fibrillation and heart failure. European Journal of Heart Failure 2013 (15) S1, S 295

In: Uric Acid
Editor: Mary Newman

ISBN: 978-1-53610-287-1

Chapter 5

TUMOR LYSIS SYNDROME

Peter L. Platteborze*, PhD, DABCC, FACB
Department of Criminology, St. Mary's University,
San Antonio, TX, USA

ABSTRACT

Tumor lysis syndrome is a rare, potentially life threatening condition that often occurs after chemotherapeutic treatment of various malignant neoplasms, especially high grade lymphomas. As the name implies, tumor lysis syndrome involves rapid tumor cell lysis which commonly results in elevated levels of uric acid and significant electrolyte imbalances. These abnormalities can result in crystal deposition in renal tubules and culminate in acute renal failure. An effective clinical management strategy is to preclude this condition by the administration of intravenous fluids and hypouricemic drugs. Historically, the drug of choice to treat tumor lysis syndrome has been allopurinol but in the last decade this has shifted to rasburicase. This recombinant urate oxidase efficiently converts uric acid to significantly more water soluble products thereby reducing the chances of acute renal failure. In 2002 this drug was approved for use in the United States by the Food and Drug Administration. Comparison studies have shown this treatment to be safer and more effective than allopurinol except for patients deficient in glucose-6-phosphate dehydrogenase where it is contraindicated. Patients treated with rasburicase need to have their uric acid levels vigilantly

* E-mail: peter.platteborze@gmail.com.

monitored and to ensure accuracy, the specimens should be kept on ice to minimize *ex vivo* breakdown.

Keywords: Allopurinol, Glucose-6-Phosphate Dehydrogenase, Rasburicase, Tumor Lysis Syndrome, Uric Acid

INTRODUCTION

The advancement of modern medicine has led to treatment options of tremendous benefit to mankind but this has on occasion resulted in new, dangerous conditions. Tumor lysis syndrome (TLS) is one such condition. Following the therapeutic administration of cytotoxic agents to destroy various malignant neoplasms TLS can develop. This occurs most often in patients being treated for highly aggressive lymphomas, such as acute lymphoblastic leukemia, acute myeloid leukemia and Burkitt's lymphoma, but has been reported in virtually every cancer type [1]. A broad range of treatments have been implicated to include cisplatin, etoposide, fludarabine, intrathecal methotrexate, rituximab, bortezomib, thalidomide, and paclitaxel [1, 2] as well as ionizing radiation, interferon alpha, and endocrine therapies involving corticosteroids, dexamethasone, and tamoxifen. Though rarely documented, TLS can also occur spontaneously [3]. With the availability of increasingly effective antitumor regimens, there is an increased likelihood of patients developing TLS.

As its name implies, TLS involves the rapid destruction of a tumor mass which commonly results in the release of intracellular components that if left untreated can cause death. Consistent with the presence of extensive cellular lysis, one often observes elevated levels of lactate dehydrogenase as well as hyperkalemia, hyperphosphatemia, and hypocalcemia in the blood. Significant amounts of nucleic acids are also released from the lysed cells and the subsequent catabolism of purines results in a marked increase of uric acid. We recently published a clinical case study that described a pediatric intensive care unit patient in the early stages of TLS [4]. This young African American male had previously been diagnosed with acute lymphoblastic leukemia and had a rapidly growing tumor mass that was obstructing his breathing. Regardless of the etiology of TLS, if left untreated it can result in extensive crystal deposition of uric acid in the renal tubules of the kidney which can culminate in acute renal failure.

It is also important to note that hyperphosphatemia can also result in calcium phosphate deposition in the tubules and that this event occurs more readily in the presence of uric acid and vice versa [3].

TREATMENT

An effective clinical management strategy is to preclude this life threatening condition by the administration of intravenous (IV) fluids and hypouricemic drugs. Pushing fluids dramatically improves renal perfusion and glomerular flow. By inducing a large volume of urine output this also limits the potential of crystal formation in the tubules. Historically, the drug of choice to treat TLS was allopurinol but in the last decade this has shifted to rasburicase. This drug is a recombinant urate oxidase that is expressed in a modified strain of *Saccharomyces cerevisiae*. Both drugs are currently used to treat TLS and each has its own advantages and disadvantages.

Allopurinol is a structural isomer of hypoxanthine that competitively inhibits the enzyme xanthine oxidase thereby blocking the natural metabolism of xanthine to uric acid. In effect, it limits the generation of new uric acid and is a relatively inexpensive generic medication that is typically orally administered. However, it does have many limitations. These include the inability to reduce any pre-existing elevated serum uric acid and it has been associated with hypersensitivity reactions such as vasculitis and Steven-Johnson syndrome. Additionally, it also has the potential to interact with a number of other drugs and it causes an accumulation of xanthine. Since xanthine is less water soluble than uric acid, allopurinol treatment may actually lead to an increased risk of crystal precipitation in the renal tubules.

Based upon these concerns, the often preferred TLS treatment option is rasburicase. In 2002 it was approved for use in children by the United States Food and Drug Administration (FDA). Seven years later the FDA approved it for use in adults.

This drug (brand name Elitek in the United States and Fasturtek elsewhere) compensates for the inability of the human body to express urate oxidase due to the presence of a nonsense mutation [2]. It is administered by IV. This recombinant enzyme efficiently catalyzes the conversion of uric acid to allantoin, hydrogen peroxide and carbon dioxide. Allantoin is a very water soluble product. In fact, it is five to ten times more soluble in urine than uric acid, thereby facilitating excretion and greatly reducing the risk of renal crystal formation.

The use of rasburicase in patients yields significantly faster reduction in hyperuricemia and supports more efficient kidney function than the use of allopurinol in comparable patients. Its judicious use in the previously mentioned pediatric case resulted in the rapid reduction of serum uric acid levels and the avoidance of acute renal injury. Rasburicase is generally well tolerated, does not react with other drugs and is considered to be more clinically cost effective despite the marketed drug being much more expensive than generic allopurinol.

While rasburicase is generally safer than allopurinol it is important to note that it is contraindicated in patients with a deficiency of the enzyme glucose-6-phosphate dehydrogenase (G6PD). The drug label contains a boxed warning to this effect. G6PD is abundantly found in red blood cells (RBC) where it maintains normal levels of nicotinamide adenine dinucleotide phosphate (NADPH) that leads to healthy levels of reduced glutathione. Individuals who are G6PD deficient are highly susceptible to oxidative damage from rasburicase generated hydrogen peroxide which can cause extensive RBC lysis and severe methemoglobinemia.

It is worth noting that G6PD is the most common type of enzyme deficiency in humans, with an estimated 400 million people affected worldwide. Further, it is an X-linked inherited disorder most commonly affecting persons of African, Southeast Asian, and Mediterranean ethnicity. In the United States, African American males are most commonly affected, with an estimated 10% affected.

A current summary of G6PD deficiency is freely available online on the American Association for Clinical Chemistry's site Lab Tests Online [5]. At least one fatality has been documented that involved rasburicase treatment of a 62-year-old African American man who was unknowingly G6PD deficient [6]. To avoid this, it is recommended that patients considered at high risk of having this deficiency have their G6PD levels measured prior to receiving rasburicase.

LABORATORY TESTING

It is essential that patients receiving rasburicase treatment have their uric acid levels vigilantly monitored to verify efficacy. Because the drug's catalytic activity continues post-collection, specimens should be tested as soon as possible, preferably within four hours [7].

Further, to ensure accurate laboratory test results, the tubes should be pre-chilled and the collected specimens immediately placed on ice to minimize *ex vivo* breakdown of uric acid [7, 8]. Patient's uric acid levels should be reevaluated four hours post-administration from the first dose and then every 6 to 12 hours until normalization occurs.

Conclusion

TLS is a potentially life threatening consequence derived from the treatment of various malignancies, especially aggressive cancers. Its incidence may increase in the future with the development of new, increasingly effective antitumor therapies.

Prophylactic treatments are available that have been proven to be very effective in preventing TLS from developing, especially the relatively new recombinant urate oxidases.

References

[1] Wilson, F. P., Berns, J. S. (2014). Tumor Lysis Syndrome: New Challenges and Recent Advances. *Adv. Chronic Kidney Dis.,* 21: 18 - 26.

[2] Davidson, M. B., Thakkar, S., Hix, J. K., Bhandarkar, N. D., Wong, A., Schreiber, M. J. (2004). Pathophysiology, Clinical Consequences, and Treatment of Tumor Lysis Syndrome. *Am. J. Med.,* 116: 546-554.

[3] Larson, R. A. and Pui, C.-H. (2016). UpToDate. Tumor Lysis Syndrome: Prevention and Treatment. Available from http://www.uptodate.com/contents/tumor-lysis-syndrome-prevention-and-treatment.

[4] Platteborze, P. L., Matos, R. I., Gido-Vandiaz, V. K., and Wilhelms, K. W. (2015). An Unexpected Emergency Request for Glucose-6-Phosphate Dehydrogenase Testing in a 9-Year-Old African-American Boy. *Lab. Med.,* 46: 150-152.

[5] Platteborze, P. L. (2016). American Association for Clinical Chemistry Lab. Tests Online. Glucose-6-Phosphate Dehydrogenase. Available at https://labtestsonline.org/understanding/analytes/g6pd/tab/test.

[6] Bucklin, M. H., Groth, C. M. (2013). Mortality following Rasburicase-induced Methemoglobinemia. *Ann. Pharmacother.,* 47: 1353-1358.

[7] Sanofi-aventis U.S. Elitek (rasburicase) Powder for Solution, for Intravenous Infusion, Section 5.4, Laboratory Sample Handling Procedure. Available from http://products.sanofi.us/elitek/elitek.html.

[8] Platteborze, P. L. and Wilhelms, K. W. (2015). Request for Uric Acid Analysis on an Iced Specimen. *Clin. Chem.,* 61: 1212-1213.

BIOGRAPHICAL SKETCH

Peter L. Platteborze

Affiliation: Department of Criminal Justice and Criminology, St. Mary's University, San Antonio, TX USA

Education: B.S. Biochemistry, University of Tampa
PhD Biochemistry, University of South Carolina
Clinical Chemistry Post-doctoral Fellowship, University of Washington

Professional Appointments: Assistant Professor, St. Mary's University

Honors: DABCC, FACB

In: Uric Acid
Editor: Mary Newman

ISBN: 978-1-53610-287-1

Chapter 6

CIRCULATING URIC ACID DOES NOT MANDATORILY DECREASE WHEN LIPID HANDLING IS IMPROVED: THE CASE OF POLYPHENOL-TREATED OBESE ZUCKER RATS

***Christian Carpéné*[1,*], *Marta Llarena*[2], *Luis Aldámiz-Echevarría*[2], *Fernando Andrade*[2], *Pauline Decaunes*[1] *and Elizabeth Hijona*[3]**

[1]Institut des Maladies Métaboliques et Cardiovasculaires, I2MC, UMR 1048 INSERM, and Univ. of Toulouse 3, Toulouse, France
[2]Division of Metabolism, Cruces University Hospital and BioCruces Health Research Institute, Barakaldo, Spain
[3]Department of Gastroenterology, Biodonostia Research Institute, University of Basque Country, San Sebastián, Spain

ABSTRACT

Uric acid is one of the purine metabolites that animals have to excrete together with other nitrogen waste products such as ammonia and

[*] Corresponding author: Dr. Christian Carpéné. INSERM U1048, I2MC, CHU Rangueil, 31432 Toulouse, France., e-mail: christian.carpene@inserm.fr.

urea. Before being eliminated, uric acid circulates in blood and may precipitate as urate crystals when its concentration increases excessively, a situation known as "gout attack". Besides its poor solubility, uric acid is a potent antioxidant in blood and should not be considered only as a potential toxic waste. Accordingly, uric acid levels change not only when nitrogen metabolism is altered but also during inflammatory, metabolic and cardiovascular diseases. Dietary polyphenols have been intensively studied in animal models of these diseases and reported to alleviate many of the complications of diabetes and obesity. The most known member of this family, resveratrol is now recognized for its antioxidant properties and for exhibiting promising beneficial effects, related to its cardioprotective, renoprotective, anti-inflammatory, antidiabetic and anti-obesity actions. However, the benefits of resveratrol are discussed regarding human health. In this context, we investigated the influence of a hydroxylated derivative of resveratrol, piceatannol, on obesity complications in an animal model exhibiting insulin resistance, dyslipidemia and early signs of nephropathy: the obese Zucker rat. We explored the changes in uric acid in conditions in which piceatannol reduced fibrosis biomarkers and lipid peroxidation in the kidney (repeated oral intake of 15 and 45 mg/kg/day for 6 weeks). Surprisingly, the renoprotective effect of piceatannol was not accompanied by a reduction of circulating uric acid, especially with the higher piceatannol dose, which increased by 30% the plasma uric acid. Both doses of piceatannol tended to decrease circulating triglycerides, and the higher dose decreased plasma non-esterified fatty acids and LDL-cholesterol while glycaemia and blood markers of glycation remained unaltered. Thus, in a situation indicating that piceatannol supplementation is improving lipid handling in obese rats, uric acid appeared to be negatively correlated with LDL-cholesterol levels and plasma triglycerides. Other analyses revealed that uric acid exhibited a positive relationship with kidney sirtuin (SIRT-1, related to antioxidant defences) and a negative relationship with kidney injury molecule (KIM-1, a marker that increases with renal dysfunction). In all, our data indicated that an improvement of lipid handling could be induced by polyphenol supplementation without lowered uricemia. This suggested that moderately increased circulating uric acid could participate to delay renal dysfunctions, although severe hyperuricemia is deleterious since involved in kidney stone formation.

Keywords: piceatannol, dietary polyphenols, triglycerides, cholesterol, kidney injury molecule, sirtuins, obesity

INTRODUCTION

In this chapter, we will focus attention on an experimental situation in which dietary-induced improvement of renal functions and mitigation of hyperlipidemia coexist with moderately increased uric acid levels. This occurs when polyphenol supplementation is given to a model of genetic obesity, the obese Zucker rat. The authors do not aim to question the clinical use of uric acid as a marker of the complications of inflammatory, metabolic and cardiovascular diseases, since they agree with the deleterious outcomes associated with hyperuricaemia. Nevertheless, regarding the complex role of uric acid in metabolic syndrome, they propose that the presence of this biomolecule in plasma, already recognized to be linked with purine metabolism, antioxidant defences and renal function, could be influenced by polyphenol ingestion.

It is widely accepted that uric acid levels do not change only when nitrogen metabolism is altered but also during inflammatory, metabolic and cardiovascular diseases such as the complications of diabetic and obese states. In fact, serum uric acid levels result from the balance between urate synthesis and excretion. The excessive consumption of fructose, increasingly present in sweetened food items and beverages, has been proposed to enhance the risk for metabolic syndrome and to induce hyperuricaemia via an intensification of purine metabolism [1]. Yet, there are two faces to the coin: uric acid is not merely a waste product of purine metabolism; it is also a systemic antioxidant. Clinical studies have elegantly evidenced that obese subjects with high circulating levels of uric acid had a greater antioxidant capacity in their serum and less oxidative stress markers than patients with lower uric acid levels. However, the obese patients with high uric acid exhibit reduced insulin sensitivity when compared to matched control [2]. Moreover, interventions aiming at lowering the hyperuricaemia of these patients increased oxidative stress but did not improve insulin sensitivity [2].

In addition to its effects on carbohydrate metabolism and on glucose tolerance improvement, insulin is also involved in lipid handling. We hypothesized therefore that an improvement of the altered lipid metabolism found in insulin-resistant obese state was paralleled with a reduction of uric acid plasma levels. Prolonged treatment with resveratrol has been described to improve lipid metabolism in the obese Zucker rat, a genetic model of hyperphagia [3]. We recently reported in the same obesity model that diet supplementation with a resveratrol analogue, piceatannol (trans-3,4,3′,5′-tetrahydroxystilbene), also alleviated various complications of obesity [4]. We therefore further studied in this model the variations of circulating uric acid in response to piceatannol. Another reason that prompted us to study the putative influence of piceatannol on uric acid is that it has been recently described to inhibit monoamine oxidase (MAO) activity, together with its parent polyphenol resveratrol [5]. At this stage, it is important to mention that MAO, as well as other amine oxidases in the organism, releases ammoniac when oxidizing its amine substrates. Ammoniac is known to alter the solubility of uric acid, an aspect that could also influence the regulation of uricaemia. Piceatannol is a natural polyphenol much less known than resveratrol, although both stilbenes are present at similar amounts in several wines [6]. Note that the structural formulae of resveratrol and its hydroxyl derivative piceatannol are available in [5], together with their docking poses in MAO enzyme and in semicarbazide-sensitive amine oxidase, another amine oxidase abundant in the adipose tissue of obese models [7].

Since we previously observed that treatment with benzylamine, a substrate of semicarbazide-sensitive amine oxidase decreased plasma uric acid and improved glucose tolerance in obese and diabetic mice [8], we expected that piceatannol supplementation could influence uricaemia in rats, either. To this aim, we measured uric acid levels after a prolonged diet supplementation with piceatannol in the obese Zucker rat, which offers the advantage to develop obesity even when fed a standard rodent chow. This avoided any change in the proportional intake of fructose, a bias that occurs when using high-fat diet or high-sucrose/high-fructose diets. In the following paragraphs, we present and discuss the results of such basic exploration.

WEIGHT GAIN AND BIOCHEMICAL CIRCULATING PARAMETERS IN PICEATANNOL-TREATED OBESE RATS

The interest of piceatannol for the metabolic and cardiovascular complications of obesity has been reviewed [6]. We have reported in a recent study the multiple actions of this resveratrol derivative in obese Zucker rats [4]. Succinctly, it can be stated that piceatannol administration under the form of daily oral gavage at 15 or 45 mg/kg body weight/day for 6 weeks (in group P15 and P45, respectively) did not limit the impressive body weight gain of the obese Zucker rat, a model of severe hyperphagia, but improved its hyperlipidemia. The reduction of the circulating levels of lipids occurred though there was no change in body weight, as the mean final body weights were comprised between 401 and 403 g for the control and the two treated groups [4].

Figure 1A shows that in the groups P15 and P45, the plasma levels of non-esterified fatty acids (NEFA), were lowered respectively to 87.0 ± 4.2% and 76.5 ± 6.4% of the control values, set at 100% ($p < 0.03$). Similarly, triglycerides were reduced to 69.5 ± 9.9% and 75.0 ± 10.4% of the control values found in obese untreated group. Total cholesterol was not depressed by piceatannol treatment, while the "bad" cholesterol transported in the LDL fraction was lowered to 78.8 ± 6.7% in the P45 group ($n = 10$, $p < 0.03$), and the "good" cholesterol slightly tended to increase up to 106%.

Of note, all these decreases of the elevated circulating lipids were not accompanied by any decrease of the fasting glycaemia. The widely recognized hyperinsulinemia of the obese Zucker rat was not modified by piceatannol treatment [4]. It must be reminded here that obese rats maintain blood glucose values within normoglycaemic range at least until the age of six months (their age at sacrifice in this study), by efficient adaptive mechanisms [9] that were not improved by piceatannol ingestion. In addition, we measured several markers of glycation (a non-enzymatic reaction of glucose with proteins, known to increase with hyperglycaemia). The glycated hemoglobine, determined in blood remained unchanged between control, P15 and P45 groups (Figure 1B). Similarly, the plasma fructosamine levels were equivalent in three groups (Figure 1B). The observed glycated haemoglobin levels were in accordance with the range of values already reported for obese Zucker rats [10], indicating that blood glucose handling was under control at the expense of a net hyperinsulinemia. Thus, the absence of change in fasting insulin and glucose levels in response to piceatannol [4] was confirmed here by unaltered process of the two blood glycation markers studied.

Although piceatannol treatment was unable to limit body weight or to improve blood glucose control in rats that rapidly become obese, it alleviated several complications of obesity, including reduction of elevated circulating lipids. Consequently, the misused term "burning fat agent" cannot be applied for piceatannol, which can be considered more simply as a "lipid-lowering agent." In other words, this food supplement could be endowed with anti-hyperlipidemic properties beneficial for the treatment or prevention of obesogenic conditions, but our study failed to evidence its putative capacity to lower hyperinsulemia or hyperglycaemia. In fact, piceatannol has been demonstrated to lowers blood glucose in other obese and diabetic models [11].

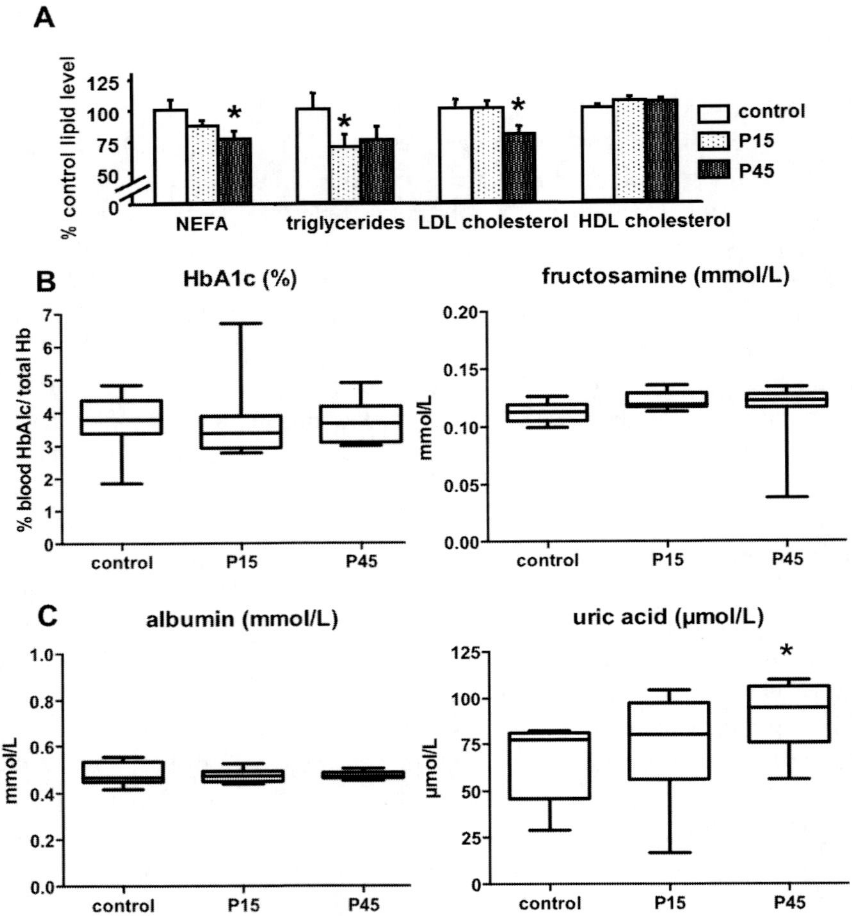

Figure 1. Circulating levels of lipids, protein glycation markers, albumin and uric acid in obese rats: influence of piceatannol oral treatment. A) Main circulating lipids are expressed as control values, set 100% reference in the untreated group of obese Zucker rats fed a standard diet (control). Mean ± S.E.M. of these percentages are given for the groups receiving daily piceatannol by oral gavage 15 or 45 mg/kg bw during 6 weeks (P15 and P45, 10 animals per group). Statistically different from control group at: * $p < 0.05$. B) The glycated haemoglobin (HbA1c) was measured in blood, while fructosamine was measured in plasma. Box and Whiskers plot is shown for each above defined group. C) Plasma albumin and uric acid in the three groups of obese Zucker rats. Statistically different from control group at: * $p < 0.05$.

Since treatments that improve blood glucose handling also reduce uric acid levels [8, 12], we asked whether piceatannol supplementation could lower uric acid levels, although it reduced circulating lipids rather than blood glucose. The study of a putative modulation of uric acid was also prompted by several aspects linking the oxidative stress of the obese Zucker rat, which exhibits early kidney lesions, renal dysfunction, supposed to be linked with hyperuricaemia. Lastly, searching for a putative modulation of uricaemia by piceatannol was justified by the fact that, while uric acid plays an antioxidant role especially in blood [2], piceatannol is also a remarkable anti-oxidant/pro-oxidant molecule exhibiting both *in vitro* [13] and *in vivo* noticeable actions on redox balance [14].

Figure 1C shows that piceatannol treatment failed to alter albumin levels in plasma. As we already reported that piceatannol did not change plasma urea levels [15], it can be assessed that piceatannol was likely devoid of deleterious effect of protein catabolism. This was in agreement with the reduced proteinuria that characterized the slight improvement of renal function by piceatannol treatment [15]. In these conditions, it was somewhat unexpected to observe that piceatannol increased plasma uric acid (Figure 1C). Nonetheless, uric acid belongs together with urea and ammonia to the family of end-products of nitrogen catabolism in animals, and it is more linked to purine metabolism than to protein catabolism. In addition to its poor solubility characteristics, uric acid is also a biomolecule with high antioxidant properties: its increase after piceatannol treatment could be considered as belonging to an overall adaptation to oxidative stress. The concern is that uric acid circulating levels have been repeatedly reported to increase with cardiovascular diseases, diabetes and obesity [16], and any elevation of its value in blood or in urine is considered as deleterious, since its excess is involved in gout attack (arthritis) or kidney stones [1, 17]. Indeed, it is far from clear whether increased uric acid is a typical marker for cardiovascular risk since this biomolecule varies with other diseases [18]. Therefore, although increased plasma uric acid and decreased uric acid clearance are supposed to be deleterious in the metabolic syndrome [19], we further compared this modulation with those of the main markers of kidney function, various indicators of oxidative stress, and circulating lipids.

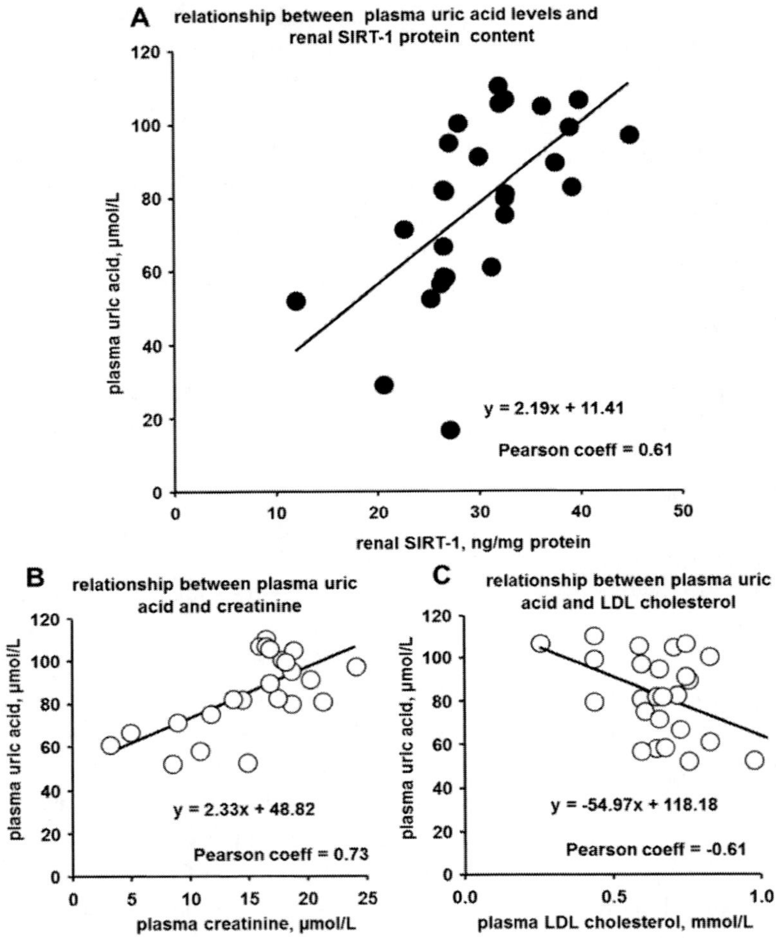

Figure 2. Relationship between plasma uric acid and sirtuin protein abundance in kidney, or creatinine and LDL-cholesterol plasma levels. Upper panel: the linear regression analysis of the relationship between plasma uric acid (on Y axis) and renal SIRT-1 protein content (X axis) led to a regression line (the equation of which is indicated under the form y = ax + b, together with Pearson's correlation coefficient ($p < 0.001$). Lower panels: Equation of the regression line (plain line) is given for the correlational plots defined by the amount of plasma uric acid on Y axis and by the circulating creatinine (left panel, $p < 0.0001$) or the LDL-cholesterol levels (right panel, $p < 0.001$) on X axis. All the studied rats, irrespective of their experimental group, were included in these analyses, save two rats characterized by low uric acid levels (detectable in the upper panel), which also exhibited abnormally low values of other plasma parameters and were considered as outliers from P15 group, thereby omitted.

COMBINED EFFECTS OF PICEATANNOL TREATMENT ON URIC ACID PLASMA LEVELS AND KIDNEY INJURY MARKERS

A close relationship was evidenced between plasma uric acid and sirtuin (SIRT-1) content in kidney when plotting the individual values of the three experimental groups of rats in the same correlational graph (Figure 2A). The more elevated was uric acid in plasma, the higher was renal SIRT-1 protein. Since both elevated levels occurred in piceatannol-treated animals, and since resveratrol has been reported to increase the expression of SIRT-1 in the kidneys of diabetic rats [20], it can be deduced from such analysis that piceatannol, like resveratrol, was activating expression and/or function of the protein deacetylase SIRT-1 involved in anti-oxidant defences and in improvement of lipid utilization [21].

In contrast, negative relationship was found between the uric acid levels and the renal abundance of kidney injury molecule (KIM-1), a marker that increases with renal dysfunction [22]: Pearson coefficient was -0.52 ($p < 0.007$) when all the three groups were treated together for correlational analyses (not shown). In fact, KIM-1 is a recognized marker that increases in many situations of renal injury and we evidenced that piceatannol-treated rats exhibited lower KIM-1 levels in kidneys and in urine [15]. Thus, increased uric acid was corresponding to an increased antioxidant status, which limited kidney injury and, in turn, repressed KIM-1 expression in kidneys. We also indicated that such signs of piceatannol-induced delay in the onset of kidney lesions occurred without change in kidney weight but with a reduction of urinary protein/creatinine ratio, indicative of an improvement of renal function. Thus, even if plasma creatinine, an indicator of kidney tubular dysfunction, was positively correlated with plasma uric acid (Figure 2B), one has to consider that the increased values of uric acid after piceatannol supplementation were associated with many other signs of improvement of renal function. Moreover, creatinine values found in the P45 group were increased by less than 20% when compared to control group (17 ± 1 and 14 ± 3 μmol/L, respectively, NS), and remained, in term of absolute values (see X-axis of Figure 2B), lower than those reported for older Zucker rat with overt renal dysfunctions (approx. 37 μmol/L between the age of 6 and 9 months) [9]. Another concern with creatinine in the Zucker rat is that plasma values are lower in obese than in lean rats [9]. The concomitant increase of creatinine and uric acid in the groups of obese rats receiving piceatannol, could be somewhat considered as a normalization towards the lean control condition. Facing to more substantial decrease of KIM-1 content in kidney and urine (both reduced by piceatannol 45 mg/kg/day from 277 ± 78 to 114 ± 49 pg/mg protein, and from 9.0 ± 2.7 to 4.5 ± 1.9 ng/mL) [15] than to the modest increase in creatinine after treatment, we assumed that piceatannol was limiting rather than accelerating the spontaneous kidney alteration occurring in obese Zucker rats even in the absence of hypertension [9]. Considering as a whole that increase in uric acid was paralleled by an increase of kidney SIRT-1 expression (Figure 2A), and a decrease of KIM-1, which in turn was associated with lowered lipid peroxidation markers in kidney (TBARS) [15], we concluded that the polyphenol was somewhat beneficial in delaying the age-dependent onset of kidney dysfunction in obese rats. Whether the uric acid increase was cause or consequence of this renoprotective effect cannot be stated at present. Nevertheless, it can be at least asserted that piceatannol was improving renal function and elevating uric acid at the same time.

Increase of Uric Acid *vs* Decrease of Lipid Circulating Levels

Figure 2C shows that a negative relationship was detected between plasma uric acid and LDL cholesterol. The piceatannol-treated rats exhibited a trend to higher uric acid values together with reduced levels of the "bad" cholesterol. Such relationship is rather surprising when considering uric acid as a surrogate marker of metabolic syndrome [16, 19]. On the opposite, a positive relationship was evidenced between plasma triglycerides and KIM-1 renal content or urine excretion (not shown), traducing that piceatannol treatment tended to decrease both triglycerides and renal or urinary KIM-1 (respective values in P45 group were 75 ± 10, 41 ± 17 and 49 ± 21% of untreated obese reference, set at 100%). Since piceatannol concomitantly increased uric acid (135 + 9%), we looked at putative opposed variations of these parameters. As in the above-depicted case of LDL cholesterol, a negative relationship was evidenced between plasma uric acid and triglycerides (equation of the regression line was: $y = -2.63x + 103$, Pearson coefficient was -0.64, $p < 0.001$, not shown). Taken together, these analyses definitely indicated that a recovery of dyslipidemia occurred without any decrease of plasma uric acid.

EXPERIMENTAL SECTION

Thirthy male Zucker rats (Crl:ZUC(Orl)-Lepr^{fa}) were handled in accordance with the European guidelines for experimental animal care and under an agreed protocol at Biodonostia Institute (#ANIM21/13).. They were housed as previously described [4] and separated into three groups: a control one and two receiving piceatannol (purity >90%, Great forest Biomedical Ltd, Hangzhou, PR China) by orogastric gavage 15 and 45 mg/kg body weight/day for 6 weeks. At the end of treatment, body and organ mass were measured after sacrifice under isofluorane anaesthesia [15] while uric acid and various metabolic parameters were measured in blood or plasma. Kidney Injury Molecule-1 (KIM-1) and other kidney markers were measured on frozen samples as previously described [15]. Assays of circulating uric acid were performed with a kit from Horiba ABX Medical (Montpellier, France) using an uricase-peroxidase-based spectrophtometric method.

CONCLUSION

Our observations indicated that piceatannol treatment exerts an overall beneficial action in obese rats, including the renoprotective, cardioprotective and antihyperlipidemic effects, already described in detail elsewhere [4, 15] while they did not reduce uric acid, as expected from any treatment alleviating metabolic syndrome. Nevertheless, these observations are not in total disagreement with the consideration of uric acid as a marker of metabolic syndrome. They merely indicate that not all the situations limiting the complications associated to obesity are accompanied with a decreased uric acid rate in the organism. At this stage, it is important to note that, even increased after piceatannol treatment, the uric acid levels we measured in obese Zucker rats (approx. 90 μmol/L) were lower than those found in other animal models of obesity, the high-fat diet fed mice (366 μmol/L) [12] or the genetically obese and diabetic db-/- mice (458 μmol/L) [8]. They were even lower than the limit of 290 μmol/L recognized to define healthy condition in humans. This consideration replaces our recent observations in agreement with the widely recognized deleterious effect of excessive uric acid in diabetes since the murine model were exhibiting overt hyperglycaemia and were clearly diabetic while the young Zucker rats are normoglycaemic. Moreover, it remains coherent that the supplementation with a dietary amine (benzylamine) triggering a glucose lowering effect was accompanied with a decrease of (elevated) uric acid, while piceatannol treatment, which did not reduce glycaemia, did not lower its abundance.

Other considerations led to suppose that special interactions might occur between piceatannol and uric acid in the view of previous reports. They are developed hereafter.

First, it has been demonstrated *in vitro* that piceatannol inhibits inflammatory responses in neutrophils that are challenged with urate crystals [23, 24]. In fact, urate crystals, that accumulate in arthritis and "gout attack" are known to increase calcium mobilization in neutrophils, together with superoxide anion production, PLD and cyclooxygenase activation and prostaglandin E_2 synthesis. A limitation of all these inflammatory reactions might occur in the piceatannol treated rats and should play a role in its beneficial action, but they hardly could modify the amount of soluble uric acid itself. Extrapolating the better handling of urate crystal by neutrophils to *in vivo* studies might indicate that the polyphenol helps the organism in safely managing more uric acid, leading to elevated circulating levels without negative consequences. The establishment of a novel setpoint between synthesis and elimination of uric acid could therefore emerge after piceatannol supplementation, leading to a limited inflammatory response, and its associated positive outcomes such as improved lipid handling.

Then, the direct interaction of piceatannol with one of enzymes that generate ammonia in the organism, namely MAO [5], led us to suppose that such issue was involved in the possible mechanisms controlling soluble uric acid levels. Such presumption was probably not relevant since the piceatannol-treated rats did not exhibit any detectable change in the activity of MAO or of any other amine oxidase found in the adipose tissue [4]. The piceatannol dose administered *in vivo* could not reproduce the amine oxidase inhibitory properties, which were observed at supramicromolar doses. It could be deduced that no subsequent change occurred in the rate of ammonia production and could alter uric acid metabolism or solubility. Thus, we did not found any rationale for explaining how the supplementation with a natural polyphenol increased uric acid levels in a model that responded by a delayed installation of nephropathy and hyperlipidemia.

At last, piceatannol is also a pro-oxidant biomolecule, able to generate radical species, especially when handled by quinone-reductases [5]. The increase of uric acid could therefore belong to an adaptative response to piceatannol administration, aiming at increasing the non-enzymatic anti-oxidant capacity in blood. Our observations are not contrasting with the consideration of uric acid as a surrogate marker of metabolic syndrome, since it can be proposed that an increase of its circulating levels, consistently reported with diabetes and obesity, might belong to a protective adaptative process rather than being deemed deleterious as it the case for severe hyperuricemia in various metabolic or genetic diseases.

Finally, our observations indicate that small increases of uric acid, a biomolecule endowed with potent antioxidant action, can be concomitant with several signs reflecting the mitigation of obesity complications.

ACKNOWLEDGMENTS

The authors acknowledge the co-workers of team 1 directed by Anne Bouloumié at the INSERM Unit 1048, Toulouse, France and those of the Dept. of Gastroenterology, Biodonostia, San Sebastian, Spain. This work was partly supported by "POLYFrEsNOL" project and RefBio french-spanish programme.

REFERENCES

[1] Johnson, R. J., Nakagawa, T., Sanchez-Lozada, L. G., Shafiu, M., Sundaram, S., Le, M., Ishimoto, T., Sautin, Y. Y., Lanaspa, M. A., (2013). Sugar, uric acid, and the etiology of diabetes and obesity. *Diabetes*, 62, 3307-3315.

[2] Fabbrini, E., Serafini, M., Colic Baric, I., Hazen, S. L., Klein, S., (2014). Effect of plasma uric acid on antioxidant capacity, oxidative stress, and insulin sensitivity in obese subjects. *Diabetes*, 63, 976-981.

[3] Gomez-Zorita, S., Fernandez-Quintela, A., Macarulla, M. T., Aguirre, L., Hijona, E., Bujanda, L., Milagro, F., Martinez, J. A., Portillo, M. P., (2012). Resveratrol attenuates steatosis in obese Zucker rats by decreasing fatty acid availability and reducing oxidative stress. *Br. J. Nutr.*, 107, 202-210.

[4] Hijona, E., Aguirre, L., Perez-Matute, P., Villanueva-Millan, M. J., Mosqueda-Solis, A., Hasnaoui, M., Nepveu, F., Senard, J. M., Bujanda, L., Aldamiz-Echevarria, L., Llarena, M., Andrade, F., Perio, P., Leboulanger, F., Hijona, L., Arbones-Mainar, J. M., Portillo, M. P., Carpéné, C., (2016). Limited beneficial effects of piceatannol supplementation on obesity complications in the obese Zucker rat: gut microbiota, metabolic, endocrine, and cardiac aspects. *J. Physiol. Biochem.*, 72, 567-582.

[5] Les Parellada, F., Deleruyelle, S., Cassagnes, L. E., Boutin, J. A., Balogh, B., Arbones-Mainar, J. M., Biron, S., Marceau, P., Richard, D., Nepveu, F., Mauriege, P., Carpéné, C., (2016). Piceatannol and resveratrol share inhibitory effects on hydrogen peroxide release, monoamine oxidase and lipogenic activities in adipose tissue, but differ in their antilipolytic properties. *Chem. Biol. Interact.*, in press, doi: 10. 1016/j.cbi.2016.07.014.

[6] Tang, Y. L., Chan, S. W., (2014). A review of the pharmacological effects of piceatannol on cardiovascular diseases. *Phytother. Res.*, 28, 1581-1588. Iffiu-Soltesz, Z., Mercader, J., Daviaud, D., Boucher, J., Carpéné, C., (2011). Increased primary amine oxidase expression and activity in white adipose tissue of obese and diabetic db-/- mice. *J. Neural Transm.* (Vienna), 118, 1071-1077.

[7] Carpéné, C., Desquesnes, A., Gomez-Ruiz, A., Iffiu-Soltesz, Z., Le Gonidec, S., Mercader, J., (2012). Long-term activation of semicarbazide-sensitive amine oxidase lowers circulating levels of uric acid in diabetic conditions. *Physiol. Res.*, 61, 251-257.

[8] Poirier, B., Lannaud-Bournoville, M., Conti, M., Bazin, R., Michel, O., Bariety, J., Chevalier, J., Myara, I., (2000). Oxidative stress occurs in absence of hyperglycaemia and inflammation in the onset of kidney lesions in normotensive obese rats. *Nephrol. Dial. Transplant.*, 15, 467-476.

[9] Albright, A. L., Johnson, P. R., Greene, S., Stern, J. S., (1994). Use of glycated hemoglobin to assess glycemic control in Wistar diabetic fatty rats and Zucker fatty rats. *Obes. Res.*, 2, 535-539.

[10] Uchida-Maruki, H., Inagaki, H., Ito, R., Kurita, I., Sai, M., Ito, T., (2015). Piceatannol lowers the blood glucose level in diabetic mice. *Biol. Pharm. Bull.*, 38, 629-633.

[11] Iffiu-Soltesz, Z., Wanecq, E., Lomba, A., Portillo, M. P., Pellati, F., Szoko, E., Bour, S., Woodley, J., Milagro, F. I., Alfredo Martinez, J., Valet, P., Carpéné, C., (2010). Chronic benzylamine administration in the drinking water improves glucose tolerance, reduces body weight gain and circulating cholesterol in high-fat diet-fed mice. *Pharmacol. Res.*, 61, 355-363.

[12] Ruweler, M., Gulden, M., Maser, E., Murias, M., Seibert, H., (2009). Cytotoxic, cytoprotective and antioxidant activities of resveratrol and analogues in C6 astroglioma cells *in vitro*. *Chem. Biol. Interact.*, 182, 128-135.

[13] Piotrowska, H., Kucinska, M., Murias, M., (2012). Biological activity of piceatannol: leaving the shadow of resveratrol. *Mutat. Res.*, 750, 60-82.

[14] Llarena, M., Andrade, F., Hasnaoui, M., Portillo, M. P., Perez-Matute, P., Arbones-Mainar, J. M., Hijona, E., Villanueva-Millan, M. J., Aguirre, L., Carpéné, C., Aldamiz-Echevarria, L., (2015). Potential renoprotective effects of piceatannol in ameliorating the early-stage nephropathy associated with obesity in obese Zucker rats. *J. Physiol. Biochem.*, 72, 555-566.

[15] Gagliardi, A. C., Miname, M. H., Santos, R. D., (2009). Uric acid: A marker of increased cardiovascular risk. *Atherosclerosis*, 202, 11-17.

[16] Tisler, A., Pierratos, A., Honey, J. D., Bull, S. B., Rosivall, L., Logan, A. G., (2002). High urinary excretion of uric acid combined with high excretion of calcium links kidney stone disease to familial hypertension. *Nephrol. Dial. Transplant.*, 17, 253-259.

[17] Kutzing, M. K., Firestein, B. L. (2008). Altered uric acid levels and disease states. *J. Pharmacol. Exp. Ther.*, 324, 1-7.

[18] Reaven, G., (1999). Syndrome X: 10 years after. *Drugs*, 58 Suppl. 1, 19-20; discussion 75-82.

[19] Wu, L., Zhang, Y., Ma, X., Zhang, N., Qin, G., (2012). The effect of resveratrol on FoxO1 expression in kidneys of diabetic nephropathy rats. *Mol. Biol. Rep.*, 39, 9085-9093.

[20] Rahman, M., Halade, G. V., Bhattacharya, A., Fernandes, G., (2009). The fat-1 transgene in mice increases antioxidant potential, reduces pro-inflammatory cytokine levels, and enhances PPAR-gamma and SIRT-1 expression on a calorie restricted diet. *Oxid. Med. Cell Longev.*, 2, 307-316.

[21] van Timmeren, M. M., van den Heuvel, M. C., Bailly, V., Bakker, S. J., van Goor, H., Stegeman, C. A., (2007). Tubular kidney injury molecule-1 (KIM-1) in human renal disease. *J. Pathol.*, 212, 209-217.

[22] Desaulniers, P., Fernandes, M., Gilbert, C., Bourgoin, S. G., Naccache, P. H., (2001). Crystal-induced neutrophil activation. VII. Involvement of Syk in the responses to monosodium urate crystals. *J. Leukoc. Biol.*, 70, 659-668.

[23] Gilbert, C., Poubelle, P. E., Borgeat, P., Pouliot, M., Naccache, P. H., (2003). Crystal-induced neutrophil activation: VIII. Immediate production of prostaglandin E2 mediated by constitutive cyclooxygenase 2 in human neutrophils stimulated by urate crystals. *Arthritis Rheum.*, 48, 1137-1148.

Biographical Sketch

Christian Carpéné

Affiliation: INSERM
Education: PhD in France. Post Doc in Spain.

Research and Professional Experience: amine oxidases, adipose tissue, obesity, diabetes, biogenic and dietary amines, polyphenols

Dr Christian Carpéné is Senior Investigator at INSERM, the French National Institute of Health and Medical Research, working in the Institute of Cardiometabolic Diseases of Toulouse, France (I2MC). He was graduated in the University of Toulouse, where he worked on the role of alpha2-adrenergic receptors in adipose tissue. Belonging to INSERM since 1983, he participated to the elucidation of the nature of imidazoline binding sites by demonstrating for the first time their functional link with hepatic and adipose monoamine oxidases (MAO). Then, he highlighted the insulin-like action that can exhibit substrates of semicarbazide-sensitive oxidase (SSAO), via the generation of hydrogen peroxide having insulin-like effect in adipocytes. He extrapolated to human the pioneering observations of the presence of an abundant SSAO activity in adipose tissue. At present, he his interested in antidiabetic and anti-obesity approaches, including exploration of the endocrino-metabolic effects of amine oxidase inhibitors and substrates, dietary amines and polyphenols and has published more than 150 articles and book chapters on the above-mentioned topics.

Publications of last 3 Years:

Harant-Farrugia I., Garcia J., Iglesias-Osma M-C., Garcia-Barrado M. J. and Carpéné C. Is there an optimal dose for dietary linoleic acid? Lessons from essential fatty acid deficiency supplementation and adipocyte functions in rats. *J. Physiol. Biochem.*, 2014, 70, 615-627.

Carpéné C., Gomez-Zorita S., Gupta R., Grès S., Rancoule C., Cadoudal T., Mercader J., Gomez A., Bertrand C. and Iffiu-Soltész Z. Combination of low dose of the anti-adipogenic agents resveratrol and phenelzine in drinking water is not sufficient to prevent obesity in very-high-fat diet-fed mice. *Eur. J. Nutrition*, 2014, 53, 1625-1635.

Carpéné M.A., Testar X. and Carpéné C. High doses of Synephrine and Octopamine activate lipolysis in human adipocytes, indicating that amines from *Citrus* might influence adiposity. In: *Citrus: Molecular Phylogeny, Antioxidant Properties and Medicinal Uses* (Khizar Hayat Editor) Nova Science Publishers, New York, 2014, 141-168. ISBN: 978-1-63117-989-1 (eBook).

Carpéné C., Gomez-Zorita S., Deleruyelle S. and Carpéné M.A. Novel Strategies for preventing Diabetes and Obesity Complications with Natural Polyphenols. *Curr. Medicinal Chemistry* 2015, 22, 150-164.

Carpéné C., Bizou M., Tréguer K., Hasnaoui M., Grès S. Glitazones inhibit human monoamine oxidase but their anti-inflammatory actions are not mediated by VAP-1/semicarbazide-sensitive amine oxidase inhibition. *J. Physiol. Biochem.*, 2015, 71, 487-496. DOI: 10.1007/s13105-014-0379-3.

Carpéné C., Hasnaoui M., Balogh B., Matyus P., Fernandez-Quintela A., Rodriguez V., Mercader J. and Portillo M.P. Dietary phenolic compounds interfere with the fate of hydrogen peroxide in human adipose tissue but do not directly inhibit primary amine oxidase activity. *Oxid. Med. Cell. Longev.*, 2016, 2016:2427618. DOI:10.1155/2016/2427618.

Carpéné C., Schaak S., Guilbeau-Frugier C., Mercader J. and Mialet-Perez J. High intake of dietary tyramine does not deteriorate glucose handling and does not cause adverse cardiovascular effects in mice. *J. Physiol. Biochem.*, 2016, 72, 539-553.

Hijona E., Aguirre L., Pérez-Matute P., Villanueva-Millán M.J., Mosqueda-Solis A., Hasnaoui M., Nepveu F., Senard J.M., Bujanda L., Aldámiz-Echevarría L., Llarena M., Andrade F., Perio P., Leboulanger F., Hijona L., Arbonés-Mainar J.M., Portillo M.P. and Carpéné C. Limited beneficial effects of piceatannol supplementation on obesity complications in the obese Zucker rat: gut microbiota, metabolic, endocrine and cardiac aspects. *J. Physiol. Biochem.*, 2016, 72, 567-582.

Llarena M., Andrade F., Hasnaoui M., Portillo M.P., Pérez-Matute P., Arbones-Mainar J.M., Hijona E., Villanueva-Millán M.J., Aguirre L., Carpéné C., and Aldámiz-Echevarría L. Potential renoprotective effects of piceatannol in ameliorating the early-stage nephropathy associated with obesity in obese Zucker rats. *J. Physiol. Biochem.*, 2016, 72, 555-566.

Carpéné C., Galitzky J. and Saulnier-Blache J.S. Short-term and rapid effects of lysophosphatidic acid on human adipose cell lipolytic and glucose uptake activities. *AIMS Molecular Science*, 2016, 3(2): 222-237. doi: 10.3934/molsci.2016.2.222.

Les Parellada F., Deleruyelle S., Cassagnes L-E., Boutin J.A., Balogh B., Arbones-Mainar J.M., Biron S., Marceau P., Richard D., Nepveu F., Mauriège P. and Carpéné C. Piceatannol and resveratrol share inhibitory effects on hydrogen peroxide release, monoamine oxidase and lipogenic activities in adipose tissue, but differ in their antilipolytic properties. *Chem. Biol. Interact.*, 2016, in press. doi: 10.1016/j.cbi.2016.07.01.

INDEX

A

D

G

H

M

N

Q

R

S

T